Arguing about Disability

Disability is a thorny and muddled concept – especially in the field of disability studies – and social accounts contest with more traditional biologically based approaches in highly politicised debates. Sustained theoretical scrutiny has sometimes been lost among the controversy, and philosophical issues have often been overlooked in favour of the sociological. *Arguing about Disability* fills that gap by offering analysis and debate concerning the moral nature of institutions, policy and practice and their significance for disabled people and society.

This pioneering collection is divided into three parts covering definitions and theories of disability, disabled people in society and applied ethics. Each contributor – drawn from a wide range of academic backgrounds including disability studies, sociology, psychology, education, philosophy, law and health science – uses a philosophical framework to explore a central issue in disability studies. The issues discussed include personhood, disability as a phenomenon, social justice, discrimination and inclusion.

Providing an overview of the intersection of disability studies and philosophical ethics, *Arguing about Disability* is a truly interdisciplinary undertaking. It will be invaluable for all academics and students with an interest in disability studies or applied philosophy, as well as disability activists.

Kristjana Kristiansen is Associate Professor at the Norwegian University of Science and Technology in Trondheim, Norway.

Simo Vehmas is Professor at the University of Jyväskylä, Finland.

Tom Shakespeare is Research Fellow at the Policy, Ethics and Life Sciences Research Institute (PEALS), Newcastle University, UK.

Arguing about Disability

Philosophical perspectives

Edited by Kristjana Kristiansen, Simo Vehmas and Tom Shakespeare

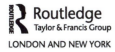

LONDON AND NEW YORK

Transferred to digital printing 2010

First published 2009
by Routledge
2 Park Square, Milton Park, Abingdon, Oxon OX14 4RN

Simultaneously published in the USA and Canada
by Routledge
270 Madison Avenue, New York, NY 10016

*Routledge-Cavendish is an imprint of the Taylor & Francis Group, an
informa company*

© 2009 selection and editorial matter, Kristjana Kristiansen, Simo Vehmas
and Tom Shakespeare; individual chapters, the contributors

Typeset in Times New Roman by
Exeter Premedia Services Private Ltd.

British Library Cataloguing in Publication Data
A catalogue record for this book is available from the British Library

Library of Congress Cataloging in Publication Data
 Arguing about disability: philosophical perspectives/edited by Kristjana
Kristiansen, Simo Vehmas and Tom Shakespeare.
     p. cm.
1. Disability studies. 2. Sociology of disability. 3. People with
disabilities – Social conditions. I. Kristiansen, Kristjana. II. Vehmas, Simo.
III. Shakespeare, Tom, 1996–
HV1568.2.A74 2008
305.9'08 – dc22
2008009464

ISBN 10: 0-415-45595-2 (hbk)
ISBN 10: 0-415-58853-7 (pbk)
ISBN 10: 0-203-89157-0 (ebk)

ISBN 13: 978-0-415-45595-4 (hbk)
ISBN 13: 978-0-415-58853-9 (pbk)
ISBN 13: 978-0-203-89157-5 (ebk)

MIX
Paper from
responsible sources
FSC
www.fsc.org
FSC™ C013985

Printed in the United Kingdom
by Henry Ling Limited

Contents

Contributors

Jerome E. Bickenbach is Professor of Philosophy and Law at Queen's University, Canada, and consultant for the World Health Organisation. His research interests include disability conceptualisation, ethics and political theory, especially theories of distributive justice.

Lindsey Brown is a researcher in Public Health Ethics at the Ethox Centre, University of Oxford, UK. Her training has been in law and she explores ethics through socio-legal and empirical research. Her research interests include health-care law, disability rights and bioethics.

Steven D. Edwards is Professor in the Department of Philosophy, History and Law, School of Health Science, Swansea University, Wales. His main research interests fall within the field of philosophy of health care, philosophy of mind and relativism.

Matti Häyry is Professor of Bioethics and Philosophy of Law at the University of Manchester, UK. He is the President of the International Association of Bioethics, and his research interests include moral theory and the ethics of genetics.

Richard Hull is Lecturer in Philosophy and Director of the Centre for Bioethical Research and Analysis at the National University of Ireland, Galway. His research interests include moral philosophy, political theory and bioethics.

Heikki Ikäheimo is a research fellow in philosophy at Macquarie University, Australia. His main fields of interest are recognition, personhood, social ontology and Hegel's theory of subjectivity.

Patrick Kermit is a doctoral research fellow at the Norwegian University of Science and Technology (NTNU). He has a degree in philosophy and is also a sign-language interpreter. In his PhD project he analyses different ethical aspects related to paediatric cochlear implantation.

Kristjana Kristiansen is an Associate Professor at the Norwegian University of Science and Technology, Department of Social Work and Health Science. Her educational background is in psychology with a doctoral degree in public health. Her research interests are in disability studies, mental health and qualitative methodologies.

Pekka Mäkelä is a researcher in the Department of Social and Moral Philosophy at the University of Helsinki, Finland. His research focuses on collective moral responsibility and the metaphysics of social reality.

Donna Reeve is a PhD student at Lancaster University, UK. She has an MA in disability studies, and her research interests include disability theory and post-structuralism with an emphasis on interdisciplinary approaches to disability.

Jackie Leach Scully is Senior Lecturer in the School of Geography, Politics and Sociology, Newcastle University, UK. Her training is in neuroscience and in philosophy. Her current research interests include disability and bioethics, the phenomenology of disability and the limits to moral imagination.

Tom Shakespeare is a social scientist with an interest in bioethics. His books include *Disability Rights and Wrongs* and *Genetic Politics: From Eugenics to Genome*. He has been involved in the UK disability movement for twenty years.

Steven R. Smith is Professor of Political Philosophy and Social Policy at the University of Wales, Newport, and is a founding member of the Newport Social Ethics Research Group (SERG). His research interests include the philosophies of disability, social justice and egalitarianism.

Berge Solberg is Associate Professor at the Norwegian University of Science and Technology, Department of Social Work and Health Science. His research interests are primarily in bioethics, especially prenatal diagnosis, the ethics of pre-implantation genetic diagnosis and the ethics of genetic databases.

Tuija Takala is Senior Lecturer in Bioethics and Moral Philosophy at the University of Manchester, UK, and Adjunct Professor of Practical Philosophy at the University of Helsinki, Finland. Her background is in philosophy, but she has also studied medical ethics and law. Her research interests include the more theoretical and conceptual issues of bioethics, such as notions of autonomy and identity.

Simo Vehmas is Professor of Special Education at the University of Jyväskylä, Finland. His training is in both special education and philosophy, and his research interests include disability theory and the ethics of disability.

Introduction

The unavoidable alliance of disability studies and philosophy

*Simo Vehmas, Kristjana Kristiansen
and Tom Shakespeare*

This book is about philosophers encountering disability and disability scholars from various disciplines encountering philosophy. The aim of this collection is quite straightforward: to provide: (1) theoretical tools for the conceptualisation of disability; and (2) well-argued and well-grounded views on definitional and normative issues for professionals and policy-makers. What makes this book novel is its focus on disability as a philosophical issue. Disability studies scholarship thus far has been mostly empirical in nature and rooted largely in sociological frameworks. Despite the in-built tendency to theorise disability in the social scientific framework, 'the development of social theory about disability is still in its infancy', as Carol Thomas (1999: 29) asserted almost ten years ago, an assessment which unfortunately still applies.

Philosophers, for their part, have usually been interested in disability in relation to major issues such as abortion, euthanasia and justice (e.g., Buchanan *et al.* 2000; Harris 1993; Kuhse and Singer 1985; Veatch 1986), but their work rarely manages to take into account larger contextual factors (social, cultural, political) that play a major part in people's disablement and which are substantial elements in the formation of the phenomenon of disability. Fortunately, philosophical contributions sensitive to the complexity of disability have begun to emerge, but mostly these contributions are focused on certain philosophical terrains, mainly ethics and political philosophy (e.g. MacIntyre 1999; Parens and Asch 2000; Nussbaum 2006; Scully 2008; Silvers *et al.* 1998; Wendell 1996).

Roughly speaking, it appears that while disability studies research has produced a highly useful reconceptualising of disability as a social phenomenon, and has produced useful empirical analyses, it lacks essential dimensions of theoretical scrutiny necessary to do justice to the complexity of the phenomenon. Philosophers, on the other hand, have traditionally been sloppy in doing their homework regarding the empirical realities and facts about disability, and have tended to treat disability in a stereotypical manner (Silvers 1998; Wasserman 2001). Yet, the conceptual and analytic rigour typical of philosophy seems to be exactly what the theoretical development of the disability research field needs. This book aims to fill this gap, providing both descriptive and normative dimensions of disability, from various theoretical and practical perspectives. We hope that the chapters in this book offer alternative and complementary viewpoints to current understandings of what disability is all about.

The present social scientific emphasis in disability research field is the result of a long historical process. Roughly three main patterns regarding disability can be traced in Western culture. The first is the *moral model of disability*, familiar from the Bible and generally the prevalent view in antiquity. According to this view, disability is a sign of the moral flaws of an individual, or his or her progenitors: for example, an infant's impairment is the result of one's parents' moral offences. If a person is impaired later in life, his or her impairment can be explained by his or her own moral failures. According to this position, disability is a disadvantageous state, usually a visible impairment, visited upon individuals (and their families) as retribution (e.g., Garland 1995; Silvers 1998: 56–9; Stiker 1999).

In the modern era, disability has been explained by scientific methods, and reduced to an individual's physiological or mental deficiencies. Disability has become, among other phenomena such as alcoholism, homosexuality and criminality, a paradigm case of medicalisation (a term which refers to a process where people and societies are explained increasingly in medical terms). The expression *medical model of disability* has become a common nickname for a one-sided view that attributes the cause of the individual's deficits either to bad luck (accidents), to inadequate health practices (smoking, bad diet), or to genes. This position views disability as the inevitable product of the individual's biological defects, illnesses or characteristics. Disability becomes a personal tragedy that results from the individual's pathological condition (Barnes *et al.* 1999; Oliver 1990, 1996; Priestley 2003; Silvers 1998).

Since the late 1960s, the one-sided medical understanding of disability has been fiercely criticised. It has been argued that medicine portrays disability in a biased manner that leads to practices and social arrangements that oppress people with impairments; interventions are aimed solely at the 'abnormal' individual while the surrounding environment is left intact. Resources are not directed at changing the environment but rather on ways to 'improve' or 'repair' the impaired individual. This is seen to lead to a social and moral marginalisation of disabled people, preventing their full participation in society. In other words, disability is a social problem that should be dealt with through social interventions, not an individual problem that is to be dealt with through medical interventions. Sociological viewpoints combined with a strong political commitment to the self-empowerment of people with impairments have become the ontological and epistemological foundation for disability studies (e.g., Linton 1998; Oliver 1996; Priestley 2003).

Indeed, the way a phenomenon such as disability is understood and explained constitutes the basis for practical interventions aimed at removing the possible hardships associated with disability. A certain view and understanding of disability inevitably directs our responses and actions. In other words, if the cause of impairment and disablement is seen to be spiritual, it is only natural to address the issue with spiritual manoeuvres, such as exorcism and faith-healing. And if disability is understood in terms of medical knowledge and is confused with impairment, then it is only reasonable to concentrate on improving a person's ability with medical interventions.

One unfortunate outcome of mechanical applications of either one of these individualistic approaches to disability has been paternalism: making decisions on behalf of others for their own good, even if contrary to their own wishes. Part of paternalism is a kind of expert system where the authorities of relevant knowledge and craft determine how the phenomenon in question should be understood and dealt with. In the religious framework, it is the clergy who are in possession of the truth; in the medical discourse, it is the doctors. In either case, the autonomy of people with impairments has too often been trampled upon, and they become merely passive recipients of the benevolent assistance provided by professionals, and other believers of the dominant disability discourse. The shortcomings of individualistic approaches to disability thus seem clear, and the emergence of a social understanding of disability has been a welcome change to disability discourse and institutional responses to disabled people's lives.

The field of disability studies has been dominated by sociology and, in the USA, also by the humanities. The research conducted is mostly empirical with the aim of verifying certain premises. For example, in the UK, disability is often seen to be a matter of oppression, and the function of research is to a large extent to clarify how people with impairments are actually oppressed. However, if disability as a social phenomenon is understood in terms of oppression and discrimination, it would seem vital to make closer analyses of concepts such as health, normality, well-being, discrimination, justice and equality – the kind of concepts that have long been discussed in philosophy. However, very little theoretical work has been done concerning the key concepts and underlying assumptions of disability studies. Hence, this book aims to contribute to the development of disability theory and a more profound understanding of the phenomenon.

Overview of the book

Philosophy examines the conceptual boundaries of human thought by means of examples and counter-examples. By rational inquiry, philosophers seek understanding about the fundamental concepts and principles involved in thought, action and reality. It is often characteristic of philosophical quests that they are undertaken for their own sake, but at the same time, it is commonly agreed that philosophising should lead to wisdom, virtue and happiness. Philosophy of disability is both substantially and methodologically a form of applied philosophy, in which philosophical theories and concepts are applied to particular circumstances and problems with practical significance, and standard philosophical techniques are used to define, clarify and organise the philosophical issues found in the phenomena under discussion. Using philosophical method in relation to practice also often has the aim of developing new conceptual tools.

Academic philosophy has traditionally been divided into metaphysics (broadly understood as including ontology, epistemology and philosophy of language), ethics, political philosophy, the philosophy of science and logic. Logic is not included in this book, and the philosophy of science is built into the metaphysics section due to its close relationship to ontology, but otherwise the structure of this book is organised on the basis of the three major branches of philosophy: metaphysics, political philosophy and ethics. These kinds of classifications are often artificial and do not do justice to the complex nature of the phenomenon of disability. Consequently, many of the chapters in this book include ontological as well as social and ethical considerations, which is understandable since these dimensions are often interwoven and cannot be properly understood as separate entities. Irrespective of some overlap, all the chapters in this book focus on analysing disability either in terms of metaphysics, political philosophy or ethics.

Part I: Metaphysics

Metaphysics consists of ontology, which is the study of the nature of existence, and epistemology, which refers to the theory of knowledge. Thus, the first part of the book focuses on examining what disability as a phenomenon is all about, and the relationship of (scientific) knowledge to the essence of this phenomenon.

The first chapter by Steven Smith in a way encapsulates this book because it discusses some fundamental ontological and epistemological ideas about disability and how they form bases for ethical convictions and social arrangements. Smith starts by discussing essentialist notions of disability that reduce the phenomenon to medically defined impairments. These accounts are based on premises that assume certain ways of embodiment and human existence as normal and desirable, or alternatively as deficient and tragic. Smith argues that these kinds of ideas are simplistic and potentially harmful in two ways: (1) they form the basis for social arrangements that exclude people with impairments from equal participation in society; and (2) they construct disability with negative meanings that undermine the subjective experiences of the well-being of people with impairments. At the same time, a one-sided social understanding of disability as well may undermine a person's identity as a disabled person if the subjective experience of impairment (e.g., pain and suffering) is ignored. Smith emphasises people's capacity for human agency, meaning that an individual may not have the power over his or her environment and various unanticipated factors, such as impairments, but a person can decide what kinds of meanings to give them and how to construe them as parts of one's personal narrative and identity. Respect for persons includes respect for subjective experiences, and this is the basis for healthy human relationships as well as fair social and political systems.

In the second chapter, Steven Edwards argues that the definition of disability is always based on some values. Whether they are medical, moral or aesthetic, conceptions about disability are connected to these values, and ultimately to some view of what constitutes a good human life. Edwards starts by analysing the meaning and significance of so-called medical values (freedom from pain, human ability, bodily form and movement) and infers that none of them is significant in their own right, but by virtue of their impact upon one's capacity to pursue the kind of projects and life one wishes to. So, at its core, the definition of disability is an ethical project and always to some extent rooted in subjective experience. Values often intertwine with each other; for instance, aesthetic tastes may affect greatly our ethical (and even medical) judgements: bodily features considered ugly and repulsive may in certain cultural contexts undermine one's moral worth. Irrespective of the value under discussion, the subjective voice of people with impairments should always be given due consideration.

In Chapter 3, Simo Vehmas and Pekka Mäkelä provide a philosophical analysis of the ontology of impairment and disability. They aim to provide a reconciliatory approach that considers both physical and social elements of the phenomenon. They also offer analytic tools for differentiating the various ontological levels that disability consists of and understanding their relationship. Following John Searle's theory, the analysis is based on the division between two categories of facts concerning the world we live in: 'brute' and institutional facts. Brute facts are those that require no human institution for their existence. To state a brute fact requires naturally the institution of language, but the fact stated is not the same as the statement about the fact. For example, the presence of an extra chromosome 21 is a brute fact, and despite of people's constructions or deconstructions, this fact remains. As for the lives of people with extra chromosome 21, social reality and human institutions then enter the picture. Vehmas and Mäkelä argue for the separation of ontological and epistemological categories where such division is in order. This is not to deny the fact that social constructs significantly shape social reality: various constructions concerning impairment and disability have considerable effects on the lives (including their narratives and identities) of people with impairments. At the same time, every socially created fact requires a physical foundation: facts exist hierarchically, and ultimately they all rest on brute facts.

The last chapter in Part I is by Jackie Leach Scully. She examines the physical foundation and the embodied nature of disability from the viewpoint of Maurice Merleau-Ponty's philosophy. Scully calls for a more nuanced and thorough understanding of the impacts of embodiment to our philosophical and normative judgements regarding, for example, quality of life, arguing that simplified conceptions about the impacts of impairments on human well-being can lead to imprudent conclusions. In line with phenomenology, she argues that a person's presence in the world is an accumulation of everyday bodily events and encounters. This being the case, a socially or biologically anomalous embodiment will inevitably affect in one way or another the nature of the everyday events and encounters because human body is the basis of the human mind; mental life is a product of the complex interaction between body and its setting. Although it seems clear that bodily differences probably have effects on cognitive processes, one should be cautious in jumping to conclusions. For example, it would be silly to infer that a person who was unable from birth to make voluntary, repeated bodily actions would also end up unable to think in ways as other people do. How exactly an anomalous body affects one's identity and sense of self is an issue that requires new and more exhaustive empirical knowledge.

Part II: Political philosophy

Political philosophy refers to philosophical reflection on how best to arrange our collective lives. In other words, what would institutionally be the best way to arrange our social life, and how can and should these arrangements be justified? Typically, political philosophers discuss the meaning and significance of, for example, liberty, justice and equality.

The first chapter in Part II by Heikki Ikäheimo unites ontology and political philosophy, including a descriptive and normative discussion about the meaning of personhood and social inclusion, and the connection between them. Ikäheimo starts by analysing rival concepts of personhood, and then, introduces an interpersonal concept of personhood that is based on people's recognitive attitudes towards one another. This general attitude is 'personifying' in the sense that someone is a person in practice only if other people recognise her or him as such, and act accordingly (namely, with respect, love and/or contributive valuing). Interpersonal recognitive attitudes and relationships are also the foundation of social life. It is not enough for our well-being and sense of worth to have certain basic rights, that is, to be included in social life institutionally. People need to be recognised as significant, individual subjects with their own characteristics, preferences and so on, in order to be persons both socially and psychologically. If one is overlooked by others as a person, one's psychological development and sense of personhood are compromised as well. Individual differences and anomalies, such as impairments, in practice often lead to non-recognition and social exclusion, or in other words, one is included in social life by others *as a non-person*. This recognition-theoretical approach poses an ethical and a political requirement to demolish degrading and exclusive attitudes and practices directed at people with impairments.

In Chapter 6, Richard Hull establishes disability as an issue of human freedom, constricted and determined by the abilities that our societies as well as our aptitudes provide us with. We are free to do something only if we are able to do it. If our inability is caused by social structures and arrangements, the society is unjust. According to negative liberty theorists such as John Rawls, sufficient conditions for freedom and justice are fulfilled if someone's freedom is not violated by another person. This approach implies that physical impairment, for instance, is a natural and an internal obstacle which reduces people's abilities, but not their freedom. Hull argues that in order to meaningfully describe something as a freedom, it has to be, at least to some extent, worthwhile or realisable. Also, both social and natural contingencies can limit our freedom and need to be taken into account in social decision-making. Certain activities are reasonably valued over others which means that freedom in itself is not the sole criterion of justice. Ensuring the access to important basic freedoms such as education, employment, leisure and social interaction, on the other hand, is a serious social and political issue because they are the kind of freedoms that are valuable as such and, also, they are necessary requirements to the enjoyment of many other freedoms.

The starting point for Jerome Bickenbach's chapter is the view of distributive justice as equality, and as a product of the way society is organised. He emphasises that inequalities between individuals may be the result of 'inner' (biological) or 'outer' (social) causes, but equality demands that only those disadvantageous differences that are caused by social and economic environments must be equalised. However, this position raises some difficult questions. For example, what kind of social failure to respond to individual differences amounts to a morally significant harm? There is no excuse for not adapting the work environment in ways that a person with visual impairment can work, for instance, as an academic, but there are very good reasons for not doing so if that person wants to be a pilot. It is reasonable, or perhaps even obligatory, to eliminate or ameliorate the impact of impairments on a person's social participation. But how do impairments differ in this respect from non-talents such as the absence of musical talent or the capacity to learn specialised employment skills? Bickenbach discusses alternative accounts aimed at solving this problem, and concludes that the distinction is made on political and economic grounds: scientific or conceptual reasons alone cannot solve the issue. He argues that the consequence of democratic equality is the maintenance of the talent meritocracy, and the inclusion of individuals with impairments into the competitive meritocracy on fair and equal basis.

The last chapter in Part II is by Tuija Takala, who discusses the significance and appropriateness of group identity by comparing two oppressed groups: women and people with impairments. Both of these groups are products of social constructs based on hegemonic categories which represent the ideal forms of humanity, namely, men and 'non-disabled'. Identification as a woman or disabled has provided individuals with membership of a group of people with a similar, socially discriminated status, and allegedly similar characteristics. This has been the foundation of identity politics which has turned out to be useful both psychologically and politically. Takala, however, argues that this political agenda has, despite its noble aims, often oppressed people into certain role expectations and has left very little room for individuality. In a sense, identity politics has sometimes trampled upon people's subjective experience by restricting them to the social roles of 'women' or 'disabled' without providing room for their varying sources of identity. As a result, women and people with impairments may have to abandon their group identities if they want to thrive as individuals, because political success purportedly demands unity of voices and the united experience of being oppressed. While communities and group identities are useful in some respects, they may undermine individual empowerment if people are not seen as individual persons, but as caricatures of the group they are expected to represent.

Part III: Ethics

The main business of normative ethics is the general study of goodness and right action.[1] In plain English, the main questions of ethics are: 'What kinds of beings should we be like?' and 'How are we to live?' Philosophical ethics thus aims to describe the best features of human character and manner in a way that could be the basis for normative rules and even law-making and jurisdiction. The majority of philosophy of disability literature is about ethics, and especially bioethics.

The relationship between bioethics and disability, in turn, has traditionally focused on killing: bioethicists have mainly discussed disability as a factor that justifies either the moral permissibility of active or passive killing of people with impairments, or the prevention of the very existence of such people (Asch 2001; Vehmas 2003; Wendell 1989).

The last three chapters in Part III deal with issues related to killing. The first two chapters discuss distinct, complex and highly debated issues of 'curing' and preventing deafness. Patrick Kermit, in Chapter 9, examines the morality of cochlear implants (a surgically implanted electronic device that provides a sense of sound to a person who is deaf or severely hard of hearing). Kermit's chapter is an examination of two normative arguments and their relationship. The first argument is the one supported by the Deaf community and based on the idea that Deaf people are primarily members of a linguistic minority, rather than members of an impaired minority in need of 'cure'. The second is the open future argument developed by Joel Feinberg (and further applied and developed by many others) which claims that every child has a right *not* to have his or her future options irrevocably foreclosed. Kermit argues that the main deficiency of Feinberg's schematic system is its dismissal of a child's right to language, which is a necessary condition for the realisation of many other rights such as the rights for social and cognitive development. And in line with Wittgenstein, Kermit argues that language is the basis of one's self-image, identity and cognition, as well as setting limits to one's existence. Consequently, the fundamental right to language is a prerequisite for being in the world. A cochlear implant, as a technical device, poses no threat to the child's future autonomy if the habilitation with the implant is carried out in a way that does not violate the child's language acquisition. In light of empirical studies, Kermit concludes that a bilingual approach which would give the child access both to hearing and Deaf culture, the best of both worlds, would be the most advantageous solution.

Matti Häyry analyses in Chapter 10 the ethics of reproductive and diagnostic techniques utilised for selecting 'deaf embryos'. In other words, if we had to choose between implanting 'deaf' or 'hearing' embryos, what would ethically be the right decision? And, to what extent should the ethical judgements guide legal judgements? Häyry proceeds by evaluating a medical view that sees deafness as a disability and a harmful condition, and a social view that denies such negative value judgements attached automatically to impairments. He argues for a non-directive compromise that recognises the strengths of both the medical and the social view, concluding that the practice is genuinely contested and that the only sensible solution is a permissive legal stand. The opposing views of disability have a tendency towards a rigid legislative stance because of the underlying moral convictions. Thus, the moral contestedness of selecting 'deaf embryos' should be fully recognised in order to make possible a desirable leniency in legal terms. Accordingly, genetic counselling should provide information to parents about both sides of the issue, and in this way be 'multi-directive'; two practitioners could try to make equally strong cases for the opposing views and create a process that could ideally become non-directive.

The next chapter by Lindsey Brown extends this discussion to the legal sphere. As Brown makes evident, law is based on social values and ideas about a certain phenomenon. Law also reasserts these ideas and values and can thus contribute significantly to the lives of people with impairments. Brown examines how disability is perceived in British law. However, the points she makes will likely apply to most other Western countries as well. A distinguishing feature in the legal discourse is its almost unconditional reliance on medical expertise and understandings of disability. Judges prefer to rely on the views of medical doctors rather than, for example, on children's nurses when evaluating a child's quality of life and, consequently, whether life-saving treatment is in the child's best interests. Brown argues that the one-sided medical understanding of disability and the reluctance to acknowledge the social factors related to the quality of life of people with impairments, have led to medical and judicial paternalism. Thus, the subjective voices of people with impairments can be overruled by the allegedly objective views provided by the medical experts, which the legal profession uncritically approves, and finally puts into practice in jurisdiction.

In Chapter 12, Berge Solberg addresses perhaps the most highly debated ethical issue regarding disability: prenatal screening and selective abortion. He especially concentrates on analysing the prenatal screening for Down Syndrome, and does so from a very critical perspective. Solberg argues that impairment such as Down Syndrome constitutes a strong identity characteristic, and therefore, prenatal screening can reasonably be viewed as an expression of oppression based on identity, and of the emergent overvaluing of intellect in Western cultures. He also contends that selective abortion has been trivialised: although abortion does not amount to killing a person, it does involve a moral cost. Solberg acknowledges the importance of parental autonomy in procreation, but is not wholly convinced that prenatal diagnostics is the only way to ensure this. For example, a proper interpretation of the battery of medical tests and scans, such as ultrasound images, requires years of advanced training. Accordingly, the more medicalised and technological the process of pregnancy becomes, the less autonomous and empowered pregnant women actually are because ultimately they are at the mercy of the expertise of doctors. Solberg calls for a balanced normative position regarding prenatal screening which would carefully consider the benefits and harms of current practices.

The final chapter by Donna Reeve applies Giorgio Agamben's theory to the social exclusion of people with impairments. The central concept in Reeve's discussion is *homo sacer* which refers to someone who is not simply outside the law and indifferent to it, but who has instead been abandoned by the law. Reeve argues that prenatal diagnosis and selective abortion represent a normative scheme of what is considered to be a liveable life, and what would be a grievable death. The law protects 'normal' foetuses after the twenty-fourth week, but impaired foetuses constitute a state of exception; killing them is justifiable and can be justified on vague grounds. Also, institutional care and enforced psychiatric hospitalisation are examples of states of exception where people's rights, more or less, cease to exist. People with psychiatric histories are often seen as dangerous and posing a threat to the population at large which makes them, in a sense, comparable to terrorists. Finally, Reeve looks at examples of psycho-emotional disablism, such as staring, name-calling and intrusive behaviour. Other people's reactions to individuals with visible impairments may have detrimental effect on their emotional well-being and can indirectly even prevent them from social participation.

Note

1 Since this is a book on applied philosophy on disability, the chapters in Part III do not discuss the other branches of philosophical ethics, namely, metaethics and moral psychology.

Bibliography

Asch, A. (2001) 'Disability, Bioethics, and Human Rights', in G. Albrecht, K. D. Seelman and M. Bury (eds), *Handbook of Disability Studies*, Thousand Oaks, CA: Sage.

Barnes, C., Mercer, G. and Shakespeare, T. (1999) *Exploring Disability: A Sociological Introduction*, Cambridge: Polity Press.

Buchanan, A., Brock, D. W., Daniels, N. and Wikler, D. (2000) *From Chance to Choice: Genetics and Justice*, Cambridge: Cambridge University Press.

Garland, R. (1995) *The Eye of the Beholder: Deformity and Disability in the Graeco-Roman World*, London: Duckworth.

Harris, J. (1993) *Wonderwoman and Superhuman: The Ethics of Human Biotechnology*, Oxford: Oxford University Press.

Kuhse, H. and Singer, P. (1985) *Should the Baby Live? The Problem of Handicapped Infants*, Oxford: Oxford University Press.

Linton, S. (1998) *Claiming Disability: Knowledge and Identity*, New York: New York University Press.

MacIntyre, A. (1999) *Dependent Rational Animals: Why Human Beings Need the Virtues*, London: Duckworth.

Nussbaum, M. (2006) *Frontiers of Justice: Disability, Nationality, Species Membership*, Cambridge, MA: Harvard University Press.

Oliver, M. (1990) *The Politics of Disablement*, Basingstoke: Macmillan.

—— (1996) *Understanding Disability: From Theory to Practice*, Basingstoke: Macmillan.

Parens, E. and Asch, A. (eds) (2000) *Prenatal Testing and Disability Rights*, Washington, DC: Georgetown University Press.

Priestley, M. (2003) *Disability: A Life Course Approach*, Cambridge: Polity.

Scully, J. L. (2008) *Disability Bioethics*, Lanham, MD: Rowman and Littlefield.

Silvers, A. (1998) 'Formal Justice', in A. Silvers, D. Wasserman and M. B. Mahowald (eds), *Disability, Difference, Discrimination: Perspectives on Justice in Bioethics and Public Policy*, Lanham, MD: Rowman and Littlefield.

Silvers, A., Wasserman, D. and Mahowald, M. B. (1998) *Disability, Difference, Discrimination: Perspectives on Justice in Bioethics and Public Policy*, Lanham, MD: Rowman and Littlefield.

Stiker, H.-J. (1999) *A History of Disability*, Ann Arbor, MI: University of Michigan Press.

Thomas, C. (1999) *Female Forms: Experiencing and Understanding Disability*, Buckingham: Open University Press.

Veatch, R. M. (1986) *The Foundations of Justice: Why the Retarded and the Rest of Us Have Claims to Equality*, New York: Oxford University Press.

Vehmas, S. (2003) 'Live and Let Die? Disability in Bioethics', *New Review of Bioethics*, 1: 145–57.

Wasserman, D. (2001) 'Philosophical Issues in the Definition and Social Response to Disability', in G. Albrecht, K. D. Seelman and M. Bury (eds), *Handbook of Disability Studies*, Thousand Oaks, CA: Sage.

Wendell, S. (1989) 'Toward a Feminist Theory of Disability', *Hypatia*, 4: 104–24.

—— (1996) *The Rejected Body: Feminist Philosophical Reflections on Disability*, New York: Routledge.

Part I

Metaphysics

1 Social justice and disability

Competing interpretations of the medical and social models[1]

Steven R. Smith

Introduction

The medical and social models of disability, whilst establishing important parameters for understanding competing interpretations of disability are now probably more accurately presented as archetypes of various discourses concerning disability, allowing for a range of interpretations between these two extremes (Shakespeare 2006). It is in this light that my chapter revisits how these models can be variously interpreted in an effort to clarify the different type of claims that can be made by the Disability Rights Movement (DRM).

Briefly put, the medical model has been commonly regarded by the DRM as an inaccurate interpretation of disability forming the basis of oppressive and exploitative relationships between non-disabled and disabled people. The argument is that focusing on individual medical conditions as the causes of disability, the medical model, first, incorrectly defines disability as a fixed condition related to the severity of a medical impairment. Second, it also incorrectly assumes that it is this medical condition, often defined as 'handicap', which inevitably causes 'dependency' between disabled and non-disabled people. So, according to Colin Barnes, the medical model links the term 'handicapped' with 'individually based functional limitations' which in turn falsely implies that: 'The impairment is permanent and that [the handicapped] will almost certainly remain dependent throughout their lives' (Barnes 1991: 2).

For the DRM, the 'social model' offers an alternative paradigm for understanding disability by identifying causes of disability within social and political domains. Therefore, the experience of disability is not reduced to a fixed medical state relating to the severity of a particular medical impairment, but rather is an experience that is dependent upon how society is politically and socially organised and structured in relation to particular medical conditions. From this vantage point, the focus for the DRM is on the 'politics of disablement' where citizenship, inclusion and the problems of accessibility and discriminatory barriers to participation, are seen as central to the struggle of 'being disabled' (Oliver 1990). That is, rather than focusing on individually based functional limitations which require treatment, adjustment or 'cure' as defined by the medical model.

These models of disability though, can still be variously interpreted. Any model, after all, whilst it might provide useful generalisations concerning the character of the phenomena being examined, is relatively abstract and still requires further more substantive interpretation if it is to be relevant to specific policy and practice. I will begin by outlining two interpretations of the medical model, with one interpretation probably lying in between the medical and social models, plus two interpretations of the social model. My main argument being that (whilst these might not be exhaustive) each interpretation has distinct implications for the way disabled people are viewed and treated.

Reinterpretations of the medical model

One objection by the DRM to the medical model is that it is based on what is seen as an essentialist notion of disability (e.g., see Swain *et al.* 2003: 98–102). This associates being disabled with fixed and essential characteristics (i.e. characteristics necessarily associated with being disabled), seen via the perspective of non-disabled people and experts, that inevitably preludes a life of personal loss or tragedy. I will call this interpretation of the medical model the 'full essentialist individual deficiency' interpretation, or FEID. The main point is that policies and practices based on FEID render disabled people as passive and powerless targets of intervention through non-disabled expertise. For the DRM, this reduces the person and his or her experience to an essentially 'abnormal' and 'lesser-than' medical condition. In respect to policy and practice, the FEID is reflected in legislation throughout the industrialised world explicitly defining people with impairments as medically 'deficient', 'sub-normal' and the like. Consequently, policies of segregation and medical treatment have been legitimated where disabled people, being seen as essentially deficient, were (and are) categorised as unable to function 'normally' and therefore requiring separated and 'special' care (see Hevey 1992). At its most extreme, FEID is found in the eugenics movement and fascist ideology of the early twentieth century, where the essential deficiencies of disabled people are seen as a threat to the 'pure race'. This led not only to impaired people being segregated from the essentially normal and ideal but also resulted in the recommendation and practice of genetic eradication and even the systematic murder of people with impairments.

However, the FEID has been, on the face of it at least, rejected by most contemporary mainstream policy-makers and replaced by more social and integrated interpretations of impairment. For example, disability in part could be seen as a consequence of deficient 'bodily structure' or function (reflecting FEID) but that these in turn are deficiencies defined in relation to complex functionings operating within a social context (reflecting more social interpretations of impairment). Assuming an interface between medical and social functionings, this leads to an interpretation of disability that moves away from the FEID recognising that an impaired person might be able to participate in mainstream society, albeit as a matter of degree. So, an impaired person might be defined as deficient because they cannot walk, but then the complex social activity of mobility can accommodate for this deficiency if the environment is made accessible to wheelchair-users. It is this latter understanding of impairment I will call the 'part-essentialist individual deficiency interpretation', or PEID. Briefly put, this assumes an impaired person is able to participate at least to some extent in social activities – that is, despite their individual medical deficiencies, and as long as the social and physical environment is changed to accommodate them. In other words, PEID still assumes that essential differences between 'the disabled' and 'non-disabled' exist, but that these differences do not mean that a disabled person cannot 'function normally' at least in certain social contexts.

The PEID, which combines or synthesises elements of the medical and social model of disability, can be found in various policies and practices and is used implicitly by the World Health Organisation (WHO) in its Second International Classification of Functioning, Disability and Health (WHO 2001). This ICF classification revises WHO's earlier definition of impairment and disability, in response to severe criticisms of the first classification by the Disabled People's International (DPI). The earlier classification was eventually published as an official WHO document in 1980 but was criticised by the DPI for focusing almost exclusively on the problems of having certain medical conditions, rather than on the problems of the social environment. The second ICF classification addresses some of these criticisms, recognising that deficient bodily function can be accommodated for socially, allowing the active participation of people with impairments.

However, this compromise between the two models is still seen as inadequate by many within the DRM. So, although the second more socially minded interpretation has moved away from the FEID understanding of individual deficiency (in that the social environment is seen in part as the problem), it still explicitly relies on a medicalised understanding of disability and so cannot avoid an essentialist interpretation of normality. Therefore, disabled people are still defined as 'problematic' because they are unable to conform to standards of normality which in turn are standards that are associated with what is seen as 'ideal' or 'best'. This understanding of 'the problem' legitimates policy where the non-disabled professional, as guardian of this normalisation process, is assumed to be the expert and therefore knows best how to facilitate better social functioning. In other words, using my terminology for these different interpretations, there are still strong echoes of the FEID interpretation found within PEID and these are reflected in contemporary policy and practice. Consequently, disabled people are treated by non-disabled professionals as if the former's experience is essentially 'lesser-than' and even 'tragic', which then legitimates the latter exercising considerable power or control over the disabled client or user. For example, according to Jenny Morris:

> Someone who is blind is thus viewed as experiencing a 'personal tragedy' and it is the role of the professional to mitigate the difficulties caused by not being able to see … [Moreover] the medical and 'personal tragedy' models of disability and the attitudes which go with them are a very important part of

the powerlessness experienced by disabled people in their relationship with those professions whose role is so important to the quality and nature of our daily lives.

(Morris 1991: 180)

Therefore, mainstream policies are recommended using the PEID interpretation of impairment that either involves non-disabled experts changing the individual deficient/tragic condition through medical intervention and/or providing rehabilitation programmes for individual and social adjustment to that condition. The point for the DRM is that these policies (despite their social leanings) usually serve to reinforce the exploitation and discrimination of and against disabled people – even if these policies involve considerable resources being redistributed from the non-disabled to meet the supposed 'special needs' of disabled people (Oliver 1996: 62–77). So, intervention strategies based on the meeting of needs (defined by non-disabled experts), whilst justified on the grounds of providing care and enhancing participation, in fact function as mechanisms of social control and serve to undermine the autonomy and decision-making power of disabled people. According to Michael Oliver, recently implemented community care policy within the UK has made:

[N]eeds led assessment the linchpin of service delivery ... however, above all else assessment of need is an exercise of power, as even the language we use to talk about the exercise shows ... The professional assesses the need of the client or 'user', as they have now come to be called. ... [Yet] various studies show that professionals have distorted or defined their needs ... The new reforms do not change this balance of power at all.

(Oliver 1996: 70)

Reinterpretations of the social model

What then of the different interpretations of the social model? Much of the DRM implicitly promotes one understanding of the social model that I will term the 'politics of disablement'[2] interpretation, or POD. Instead of medical or rehabilitation polices being recommended via the FEID or PEID interpretations, attention is directed by the POD interpretation toward changing the social and political environment. In other words, this interpretation offers a structural, as distinct from an individual account of disability, in effect bracketing the personal experience of disability, other than what an impaired person might experience in relation to the social and political environment. It is via this POD interpretation that the DRM makes a clear distinction between 'impairment' and 'disability'. So, impairment is associated with a particular medical condition, which may (or may not) lead to a disability, with disability being associated with various social and political restrictions often (but not always) imposed upon people with impairments. For example, according to the Union of the Physically Impaired Against Segregation (UPIAS):

Impairment is the functional limitation within the individual caused by physical, mental or sensory impairment.

Disability is the loss or limitation of opportunities to take part in the normal life of the community on an equal level with others due to physical and social barriers.

(UPIAS 1976; see also Bickenbach 1999: 1173–86)

Following from this distinction, disability is therefore seen by many within the DRM as a thorough-going social and political concept and so should have no medical or individualised import whatsoever. So, according to Liachowitz:

Disability exemplifies a continuous relationship between physically impaired individuals and their social environments, so that they are disabled at some times and under some conditions, but are able to function as ordinary citizens at other times and other conditions.

(Liachowitz 1988: 2)

However, my argument is that the POD interpretation, although in many ways radically challenging to the two medical model interpretations, still adheres to the same essentialist myth of 'ordinary' or 'normal living', because it too relies on fixed assumptions concerning the 'normal' and 'abnormal' as related to 'ideal' and 'non-ideal' states of being. In short, the value of functionality as related to notions of ordinary citizenship is abstractly reified by the POD interpretation as a fixed ideal. That is, an ideal based on a normalised shared social goal for all individuals, including people with impairments. Of course, understandings of normalisation are conceptualised differently by the POD (compared with the medicalised interpretations above) as it refers solely to the social rather than medical origins of deficiency. However, my principal point is that all these interpretations define 'deficiency' as a 'social problem' with the ideal condition of ordinary citizenship being promoted as the main aim of each. So, the POD interpretation often portrays disabled people as looking forward to, and struggling for, a future where they can participate in the same ideal and normal state as 'the non-disabled' already are, supposedly, enjoying. For example, the ideal of 'independent living' is often promoted within the DRM as a goal for disabled people, intended to reflect characteristics of normal or ordinary citizenship. However, having this goal ignores how, in the process, rigid demarcations are made between 'normality' and 'abnormality' and between 'independence' and 'dependence' that are themselves essentialist. So, these demarcations assume falsely that (a) it is necessarily the case that all non-disabled people are independent, and (b) the condition of independence is, in any event, a desirable 'state of being' (see also my arguments in Smith 2001b: 579–98). Consequently, although according to the POD interpretation a disabled person's inability to achieve the goal of independence is related to social causes, it is still axiomatically assumed it is a deficiency that this goal remains unachieved.

To summarise, with all the interpretations of disability examined so far, the problem of deficiency is fixed in relation to essential facts (whether social, medical or a mixture of both) and that these 'facts' cause the problem. Moreover, it is a problem that is fixable through strategies that promote ordinary citizenship, whether via social and/or medical adjustment (as with PEID and POD), or, as with the FEID interpretation, with the segregation or eradication of people with impairments.

There is though at least one other interpretation of the social model that I believe complicates any exegesis of the DRM's political demands. In this interpretation, it is not only that disability is socially caused by inaccessible and discriminatory social environments but also that disability is 'socially constructed'. That is, the definition and social meaning given to individual deficiency or dysfunction (and their opposites 'talent' and 'capability') can also be conceived as related to particular social and political processes. Therefore, disabled people are discriminated against via two types of social and political processes: first, and reflecting the POD interpretation above, by social and political structural environments that exclude individuals with certain medical conditions; and second, by social and political discourses that defines what are in the first place talents and handicaps. It is this second type of social process that I will now explore, leading to what I call the 'social construction of disablement' interpretation of the social model, or SCOD.

With the SCOD interpretation it can be seen that the DRM focuses not only on issues of inaccessibility and social inequality, but also on questions concerning the negative social construction of disabled people's individual and group identity. For example, the medicalised assumption that the experience of impairment is a tragic personal loss is wholeheartedly rejected by the DRM, partly for the structural reasons explored above regarding the unequal power relationships between non-disabled professionals and disabled clients and users, but also because a disabled person's identity as a disabled person is undermined as a result. So, according to Swain *et al.*, 'for many disabled people, the tragedy view of disability is in itself disabling. It denies the experience of a disabling society, their enjoyment of life, and even their identity and self-awareness as disabled people' (2003: 71).

Regarding the discussion here concerning the social construction of 'deficiency' or 'dysfunction' (and their opposites 'talent' and 'capability'), there is a lack of recognition in respect to positive aspects of a disabled person's identity as related directly to their impairment. I will now explore how this lack of recognition can be understood in two distinct ways. First, aspects of the disabled person's identity that might be defined as talented, but occurring separately to an individual impairment, are ignored. This is relatively easy to comprehend. For example, Stephen Hawking has severe physical impairments which, according to the POD interpretation of disability, may or may not lead to a disability depending upon the social environment's accessibility. Nevertheless, whatever the impact of the social environment on his experience of disability, these physical impairments are separate from his talent for understanding maths and physics. For the DRM, disabled people's talents are often masked by dominant medical interpretations of their impaired condition (as reflected in the FEID and PEID above) which in turn lead to misjudgements about a particular disabled person's other talents or capabilities. More formally, a fallacy of composition has taken place, where a false conclusion is drawn about the whole person based on features of her constituent parts. Indeed, recognising this as a fallacy has now been accepted by mainstream policy-makers and governments who have, for example, sought to encourage and even ensure that employers think of disabled people as having talents (despite their medical impairments) through implementing various forms of anti-discrimination legislation.

However, there is a second much stronger claim that can be made using the above SCOD interpretation of the social model. A particular medical condition, considered an impairment in some respects, may nevertheless be viewed as an unrecognised talent in other respects. The problem, according to this claim, is that the 'individual deficiency' axiom found in FEID and PEID starts with what appears as a closed tautology. That is, medical impairments in all respects necessarily signify a reduction of talents for an individual who possesses them. Following those within the DRM who promote the SCOD interpretation, this is only true through a spurious definitional process. According to SCOD, the assertion that certain medical conditions necessarily signify deficiency in relation to a person's experience and self-development is itself disabling. For example, the images of disabled people as tragic victims leading unfulfilled lives tend not only to reinforce limited expectations of what disabled people might do and achieve, but also to undermine any positive evaluation that might be made about having particular conditions of impairment. The problem is that the medical interpretations of impairment do not allow for this type of evaluation as it reduces the individual and the condition to highly narrow and disabling definitional categories. Whereas, the SCOD interpretation of disability unashamedly allows and encourages a disabled person to have a positive attitude to herself, her identity and her impairment, by in effect conceptualising the latter as a positive part of that person's identity. To put it another way, possessing an impairment is in at least some ways something a person can be glad to have, and therefore is seen less as a handicap and more as a talent. I will argue below that once this more complex response to disability and impairments is understood, which permits the notion that having an impairment in certain respects at least may also signify talent-possession, then the possibilities of understanding 'impairments' in new and enabling forms are allowed. However, before exploring this claim further, Table 1.1 summarises the four interpretations of the medical and social models thus far outlined.

Impairment viewed as talent?

It is important to highlight that talents (however they are conceived substantially) are qualities or characteristics that can only be talents if not everyone possesses them to the same degree. Therefore, talent is associated with the differences between human beings rather than with their similarities. The question then is how do we value these differences including those that relate to physical and mental characteristics? Physical and mental differences between individuals might

Table 1.1 Interpretations of the medical and social models

	Interpretation	Understanding of disability
Medical models	1. full-essentialist individual deficiency interpretation (FEID)	Disability is caused by fixed medical characteristics that inevitably prelude a life of deficiency and 'abnormality'.
	2. part-essentialist individual deficiency interpretation (PEID)	Whilst disability is caused by the above medical characteristics, these can be partially alleviated by changes in the social environment, so as to enable some degree of 'normal living'.
Social models	3. politics of disablement interpretation (POD)	Disability is caused by social practices that systematically exclude impaired people from the activities of 'normal citizenship'.
	4. social construction of disablement interpretation (SCOD)	Disability is caused by the way impairments are defined and associated with characteristics that are necessarily assumed to have a negative impact on personal identity, development and fulfilment.

indicate the existence of talent if these differences are seen as having the potential of producing certain valuable forms of self-development that cannot be reproduced if there were no such diversity. If this point is conceded, certain medical conditions (whilst in some respects might be seen as a medical impairment) could be regarded as a talent in other respects.

Indeed, I would argue that this conception of medical impairment is often promoted implicitly within the DRM. For example, Jenny Morris in her book *Pride Against Prejudice* cites various disabled interviewees who see their medical condition as a source of strength and personal insight or development which would not have been achieved without having that condition. So, according to one disabled woman: 'Not all of us view our disability as the unmitigated disaster and diminishment that seems expected of us ... [For me] it has brought spiritual, philosophical and psychological benefits' (Morris 1991: 187). She continues:

> If we can appreciate that to be an outsider is a gift, we will find that we are disabled only in the eyes of other people, and insofar as we choose to emulate and pursue society's standards and seek its approval ... Once we cease to judge ourselves by society's narrow standards we can cease to judge everything and everyone by those same limitations. When we no longer feel comfortable identifying with the aspirations of the normal majority we can transform the imposed role of outsider into the life-enhancing and liberated

state of an independent thinking, constantly doubting Outsider who never needs to fight the physical condition but who embraces it. And by doing so ceases to be disabled by it.

(ibid.: 187)

There are three main points that require emphasis here and relate to the arguments above concerning how the medical and social models are variously interpreted. First, underlying her claims is the assertion that the talent is not the ability to produce these characteristics despite the medical condition (as with the FEID, PEID and POD interpretations), but rather that these characteristics are produced because of it. In other words, the condition is not a deficiency but a talent that is exploitable, given that it can lead to these diversities in characteristics and life insights. Second, these qualities underpin a much more inclusive and, by the interviewee's standards, a much richer society than exists now. This type of society would construct the concepts of normality and abnormality as merely statistical trends and not (as presently) to prelude erroneous value judgements about the diminished capability of persons with characteristics outside of these norms. Third, using the SCOD interpretation of disability, certain physical and mental conditions (usually defined as impairments) can be defined as talents because (a) they can be of benefit to the individual possessing these conditions, and (b) that this is appreciated and is of benefit to those without the condition. In respect to (b), for example, the capacity non-disabled people have for being liberated from conventional norms might be assisted by the particular insights gained by the disabled person above, who through her more immediate experience of being 'an outsider', is able to convey new possibilities for living unconstrained by these norms.

However, I will now explore the SCOD a little further, my main argument being that despite (or perhaps because of) its promising anti-essentialist credentials and more empowering interpretation of the social model, it is, I believe in serious danger of losing plausibility in respect to its understanding of the experience of some impairments. Certainly, by itself having a physical condition outside of a norm does not determine whether it is defined as a handicap or a talent. For example, a person's physical condition of abnormal tallness, although might signify a handicap in some social contexts (e.g. for being a jockey or ballerina) may be highly valued in others, in order to become, say, a much appreciated, and very well-paid, basketball player or super-model. So, the social construction process in relation to this abnormal characteristic at least, although it defines it as a handicap in certain social contexts, defines it as a talent in others. However, the social 'transferability' from handicap to talent is much less possible for the above disabled interviewee. Her abnormal characteristics are regarded as less than ideal because they are defined by others as handicaps across a number of different social domains. Therefore, although she is able to exploit her abnormal 'gift' in order to become a more liberated person and independent thinker from her perspective as disabled person, this aspect of her experience would not usually be appreciated as talent-possessing by non-disabled people. According to the SCOD interpretation, it is precisely because of these disabling social construction processes that allow others (namely non-disabled people) to define her physical characteristics as handicap across these various social domains.

However, one objection to the above move is to claim that there are bound to be abnormal medical conditions (usually defined as deficiencies) that even in principle are not subject to this type of SCOD transferability of talents and handicaps. For example, chronic incontinence might be thought of as a deficiency for all humans regardless of particular social arrangements and social construction processes. Similarly, those with severe learning impairments in any society possessing more than a basic level of technology may also be thought of as an unmitigated disadvantage for the individual concerned. Nevertheless, I would argue that even with these extreme examples, the objections to the SCOD interpretation are proceeding too quickly, and moreover are in part based on how we understand human agency and the positive responses that might be made to any human experience, despite the wholly negative views that might be held by others of these experiences. But I will now explore how this haste is in part a result of ambiguities concerning what the SCOD interpretation so far conceived is claiming, which then I believe lead to questions concerning the plausibility and coherency of the DRM's case which promotes both the POD and SCOD interpretations of the social model.

Identity and human agency

First, there are deeper political and philosophical questions for the DRM concerning how to fully embrace existing identities (reflecting SCOD) given the presence of disabling social and political structures (reflecting POD). The point being that, according to the SCOD interpretation, positive self-awareness is paradoxically worked out within a disabling social and political environment, and so to some extent at least is informed by that environment. However, if one is to take either the POD or SCOD interpretation seriously (i.e. emphasising the profound influence of society on the experience of 'being disabled'), the correlate to the latter's structural transformation (as promoted by POD) is that former positive identities (as promoted by SCOD) will presumably change in response, as the structure of society changes. Recognising this change as a social and political process therefore produces a coherency problem, between, on the one hand, the promotion of disabled identities as these exist at present, and the promotion of future non-oppressed identities as these would exist after social and political transformations have taken place, on the other.

In order to address this coherency problem, I will first separate out two claims that could be made by proponents of the SCOD interpretation, which I believe can give an added nuance to the DRM's position:

1. An individual medical condition when defined as deficient is socially constructed in every sense.
2. Medical model interpretations of disability socially construct incorrectly medical impairments as deficient in every sense.

A SCOD interpretation of the social model of disability may make both claims but this is not logically necessary. So, by maintaining a distinction between these two claims it is possible to concede some limited ground to the medical model (through rejecting the first claim) and therefore admit that having certain medical impairments at least in certain respects is deficient (in a non-social sense), albeit these are deficiencies reinforced and compounded by discriminatory social practices. Nevertheless, via the second claim it is possible to argue from the SCOD interpretation that having even a severe impairment is not necessarily an unqualified deficiency, because advantages too might be gained from having the condition, that in turn contribute to a disabled person's positive sense of her own identity as this exists presently.

I would argue that this move that combines the second social constructionist claim of SCOD with the social structuralism of POD is broadly consistent with the UPIAS distinction highlighted above between impairment – defined as a limiting medical condition: and disability or handicap – defined as a socially imposed restriction upon the impairment. Moreover, if impairment is in some sense seen as limiting according to UPIAS, it also in principle allows for some elements of the PEID interpretation of impairment.

However, is logical coherence between these various interpretations of disability (despite the appeal of theoretical elegance) what we want, either politically or philosophically? I have so far argued that these interpretations are consistent with many of the claims made by commentators from the DRM. Briefly put, the discriminated position of 'the disadvantaged' (in this case disabled people) is not only caused by social and economic structural injustice. It is also caused by what might be termed identity exclusion – i.e. when the diversity of the responses to the experiences of 'the disadvantaged' are effectively ignored or marginalised in favour of more dominant constructions.

Nevertheless, implicit within the above is, I believe, a particular conception of individual agency, the presence of which produces what I will call a 'productive tension' when understanding just human relations. This tension reflects the idea that individuals are unbound by contingent-determinism (whether social or medical), but at the same time upholds a critique of social structures that systematically excludes people with medical impairments. More specifically, what is this conception of human agency?

My main claim is that the capacity for human agency, involves what might be termed an active engagement with experiences; that is, providing individuals with the ability to step back from their circumstances and conditions and so respond to them, often in a surprising way. This surprise is born from human agency itself, based on a capacity a person has to choose her life and more importantly perhaps a perspective on her life, which is both dynamic and unpredictable. Given this capacity, an agent is able to radically go against expectations in respect to her own individual responses to her experiences and circumstances – i.e. expectations reflected, not only via dominant social norms, but from reflections of others close to her, and even perhaps from herself. Recognising this capacity, I believe has profound implications for how we understand matters relating to disability, and are reflected in the arguments presented so far.

For example, take the experience of human suffering (either physical or emotional) which may be brought about by circumstances which are beyond a person's control. The person who is suffering might wholly regret the experience and the circumstances which caused it, so leading to an unqualified deficiency in her life, as measured against, say, her understanding of personal well-being. So, to use the language of the SCOD interpretation explored above, the suffering therefore produces a deficiency in every sense. Now, it may well be that some disabled people respond to their impairment in precisely this way, and consequently conform entirely to the expectations of the FEID interpretation of the medical model. However, many other disabled people do not, and, following the SCOD interpretation, would radically reject these expectations. Indeed, there has been fierce debate within the DRM as to whether this personal perspective on disability, which views having particular impairments as deficient in every sense, should be seen as merely a product of dominant medical constructions of disability that define being disabled as necessarily tragic, or whether it is a perspective that should be taken more seriously as a legitimate response to certain conditions of impairment (see e.g. Morris 1991). There is insufficient space to explore these debates further here. Suffice it to say that my preference for claim two above of the SCOD interpretation, would allow disabled people to legitimately regret at least some aspects of their experience of impairment, without concluding that they are merely capitulating to medicalised constructions of disability.

I will now briefly outline how it is in this latter context especially that my claims about human agency can be better understood. First, it might be argued that pain and suffering (physically or mentally), although a reality that some disabled people experience, are certainly not the case for all. Pain-free impairment does not therefore lead to a reduction in personal well-being, even if it is assumed that personal well-being is necessarily threatened by the experience of pain and suffering. Second, I would contend that even the experience of pain and suffering is not straightforwardly deficient for reasons to do with the complex and paradoxical way human beings value their lives, and as related to their capacity for agency in the way I have described it. So, a person often responds to and learns from all her experiences which may include at least some level of pain and suffering, leading to a more enriched life, all things considered. It is in this context that whilst it might be thought reasonable that no-one would want a painful life, a completely painless existence could also quite plausibly be seen as deficient for most people. My further contention is that this understanding of pain and suffering, as related to the capacity for human agency, allows for a more nuanced interpretation of human experience than either the medicalised or social model interpretations so far explored. It clearly blocks any reductionist interpretations of disability, that having an impairment necessarily preludes a life that is essentially tragic. However, this understanding also prevents the tendency in certain SCOD interpretations of disability (i.e. those that make the first claim above) to deny the experience of pain and suffering for some disabled people. Nevertheless, acknowledging the force of SCOD, also allows us to recognise that having a painful impairment is not necessarily an unqualified deficiency for the individual concerned, because advantages too might be gained from having the condition, that in turn contribute to a disabled person's positive sense of her own identity as this exists presently.

Conclusion: selfhood, disability and social justice

Where do the above claims about disability and human experience more generally take us? It must be admitted that these beg numerous philosophical questions concerning, for example, the nature of 'the self' and how the thinking or reflecting subject might be perceived in relation to choices and plans and what is even meant by the phrase 'having choices and plans'. Many of my arguments presented in this chapter depend in part at least on the answers to these questions that are for now being bracketed. Nevertheless, by way of conclusion I will now pay further attention to the nature of 'the self' (for both disabled and non-disabled people) as related to the capacity humans have to go against expectations in respect to their experiences.

When experiences radically change our lives, we are often surprised by our reactions because they go against our imagined expectations. But what is meant by 'going against' in this context? What is being resisted or opposed exactly and how does this resistance relate to an imagined life, as distinct from a real life? One perhaps more obvious answer to these questions is that the 'going against' reveals inconsistencies between what a person imagines what she would do and/or be, and what she actually is or being. In other words, the going against is an epistemological problem, with the remedy being to ensure she knows herself better through personal introspection, therapy and the like. However, another perhaps less obvious answer as to what is meant by 'going against' is that, rather than revealing problematic inconsistencies in the imagined knowledge and actual knowledge of oneself, it reflects the way individual personhood is in a state of flux that changes whilst experiences are occurring. To borrow the language of existential philosophy, the self is therefore not a fixed entity or essential being that is 'back there' introspecting, but rather is a non-essential 'becoming'. More succinctly, the self is not so much known through the introspection of life but created through an active engagement with life. But how do these answers to the question of human identity relate to the arguments explored in this chapter?

To recall, according to the SCOD interpretation of the social model, the unequal position of 'the disadvantaged' is not only caused by social and economic injustice, as the POD interpretation would have it. It is also caused by what might be termed identity-exclusion. In respect to the conception of agency explored, this exclusion process occurs when diverse responses to the experiences of those defined as disadvantaged are effectively ignored or marginalised in favour of more dominant constructions. Following from the above, agent-based respect has consequently been sidelined, where a person with conditions associated with suffering is effectively reduced to a tragic and passive victim of circumstances and experiences beyond her control.

To summarise, I therefore support a particular conception of individual agency that produces a 'productive tension' when considering socially just human relations. More specifically, this tension (a) enables agents to imagine and identify with others who are creatively responsible-subjects, engaging with their experiences in highly unpredictable but often positive ways, but where (b) some subjects (in this case impaired people) might also reasonably expect a structural transformation of the social and political environment, so as to accommodate the negative consequences of having a particular medical condition. That is, even if the person experiencing this condition is happy or fulfilled with her life as it is now. In other words, and using the language of liberal egalitarian political philosophy, respecting persons as free and equal agents is central to establishing healthy human relations, recognising that social and political systems ought to re-distribute and re-structure resources to those defined as 'worst-off' but also acknowledging the human capacity for creating a positive identity whatever has been experienced. The difficult job for social and political movements, as well as liberal egalitarian political philosophy, is responding to both injunctions but recognising that these often pull in opposite directions.

Notes

1 This chapter whilst containing much original material also draws on previously published work, most particularly, Smith (2001a: 19–37) and Smith (2005: 554–76). A first draft was also presented to the University of Brighton's Centre for Applied Philosophy, Politics and Ethics conference 'Medicine and the Body Politic' in September 2006. I would like to thank very much the conference participants for their contributions.
2 This term (alongside the terms medical and social models of disability) was first used by Michael Oliver in 1990 in *The Politics of Disablement: Critical Texts in Social Work and the Welfare State.*

Bibliography

Barnes, C. (1991) *Disabled People in Britain and Discrimination,* London: Hurst and Calgary.
Bickenbach, J., Chatterji, S., Badley, E. M., and Ustun, T. B. (1999) 'Models of Disablement, Universalism and the International Classification of Impairments, Disabilities and Handicaps', *Social Science and Medicine,* 48: 1173–86.
Hevey, D. (1992) *The Creatures Time Forgot,* London and New York: Routledge.
Liachowitz, C. H. (1988) *The Social Construction of Disability,* Philadelphia, PA: University of Pennsylvania Press.
Morris, J. (1991) *Pride Against Prejudice,* London: Women's Press.
Oliver, M. (1990) *The Politics of Disablement: Critical Texts in Social Work and the Welfare State,* Basingstoke: Macmillan.
—— (1996) *Understanding Disability: From Theory to Practice,* Basingstoke: Macmillan.
Shakespeare, T. (2006) *Disability Rights and Wrongs,* London and New York: Routledge.
Smith, S. R. (2001a) 'The Social Construction of Talent: A Defence of Justice as Reciprocity', *Journal of Political Philosophy,* 9: 19–37.

—— (2001b) 'Distorted Ideals: The "Problem of Dependency" and the Mythology of Independent Living', *Social Theory and Practice: An International and Interdisciplinary Journal of Social Philosophy*, 27: 579–98.

—— (2005) 'Equality, Identity and the Disability Rights Movement: From Policy to Practice and from Kant to Nietzsche in More than One Uneasy Move', *Critical Social Policy*, 25: 554–76.

Swain, J., French, S. and Cameron, C. (2003) *Controversial Issues in a Disabling Society*, Buckingham: Open University Press.

Union of the Physically Impaired Against Segregation (UPIAS) (1976) *Fundamental Principles of Disability*, London: UPIAS.

World Health Organisation (2001) *International Classification of Functioning, Disability and Health*, Geneva: WHO.

2 Definitions of disability
Ethical and other values

Steven D. Edwards

Introduction

This chapter attempts to illustrate some aspects of the relationship between disability and values, drawing upon claims made by four notable commentators which highlight the apparently intimate connection between values and conceptions of disability. I will try to show that conceptions of disability connect up ultimately with some view about what counts as a 'good human life'. Lastly, I call into question a strong claim advanced by Engelhardt (1996) concerning what he terms 'deformity'.

There are at least two reasons for highlighting the place of values in the context of understanding disablement. The first would be to remind us that the concepts employed to distinguish among groups of people are not purely scientific, descriptive concepts, but have a value-based dimension (see Vehmas 2004). Of the approaches used in defining disability considered in this chapter, all can be shown to presuppose values, albeit explicitly or implicitly. The second reason for focusing on values is that recognising the place of values in the context of disability leads us to two questions: 'What kinds of values?' and 'Whose values are most important?'

In this chapter, I explore three types of value sets: medical, moral and aesthetic. I intend to show that differences of opinion exist in relation to the question of whose values are deemed most important in questions surrounding the issue of disability. To show conclusively that the opinions of one group count for more than the views of another is a difficult if not impossible task; and it is not appropriate to engage fully in that here. But what I present does go some way toward supporting a position where the opinions of disabled people themselves have more moral weight than the views of other parties when it comes to central questions such as the characteristics and responses to disability (Vehmas 2004). To say this, of course, is not to say that such opinions are infallible. The position just described is distinct from a crude form of subjectivism, the question of whether or not a person is disabled is determined *solely* by him or her.

Lastly, a terminological point: One of the commentators (Nordenfelt) I consider uses the term 'handicap' in his work. Apparently the term does not convey the pejorative connotations in Swedish that many find in its use in English. I have followed the author in his use of the term.

Four views

Here are some ways in which various kinds of values are prompted when considering the notion of disability:

1. H.T. Engelhardt: 'we encounter disease, illnesses, [and] disabilities ... through a web of important non-moral values' (1996: 206). Also: 'to see a phenomenon as ... a disability is to see something wrong with it' (Engelhardt 1996: 197).
2. John Harris views disability as a 'harmed condition', one 'we have a strong rational preference not to be in' (2000: 97).
3. Lennart Nordenfelt writes: the very classification of a person as handicapped 'presupposes an ethical or political decision' (2000: 123).[1]
4. Alison Lapper: 'The sculpture makes the ultimate statement about disability – that it can be as beautiful and valid a form of being as any other' (Ouch! 2005). She is speaking about a statue of herself displayed in Trafalgar Square in London.

In these quotes, I would claim that the values inherent in works by Harris and Nordenfelt are moral values, whereas those raised by Lapper's remark are aesthetic values. I return to these three value sets but begin by examining more closely the values espoused by Engelhardt which he terms 'non-moral' values.

Medical values

The values initially raised by Engelhardt he claims are 'non-moral'. And although he takes aesthetic values to have their origins in medicine ('deformity and dysfunction are ugly' (1996: 206)), he suggests there is a class of values which are neither moral nor aesthetic but which 'reflect ideals of freedom from pain, of human ability, and of bodily form and movement' (1996: 206).

Interestingly, Engelhardt refrains from attaching a name to this class or set of values. Yet he is explicit in stating that they are distinct from moral values and also from the kinds of aesthetic values prompted by works of art. And since these remarks are made in the context of his discussion of disease and value judgements, it is reasonable to infer that, if pressed to assign them a label, he would quite likely regard them as medical values.

So, following Engelhardt's discussion, one might then expand the class of values beyond moral and aesthetic to also include medical values. These values would be manifested in medical actions and their aims, such as the relief of suffering, maintenance of bodily form and movement. To expand this somewhat, with regard to suffering, it is plausible to view the relief of suffering as a central goal of medicine. Why is this? Well, suffering is a state most of us prefer to avoid, and if we are suffering, we are pleased to be relieved of it. (Of course our focus here is on suffering which the person would prefer not to be enduring, not suffering *per se*.) Suppose certain physical changes become associated with the experience of suffering, such as broken bones or bites from wild animals. These physical changes then become the focus of the medical enterprise. The physical changes themselves are not intrinsically bad, but they are devalued because they cause suffering, impede mobility, and so on. As Engelhardt states, 'clusters of value judgements make conditions stand out as problems to be treated' (1996: 205). A similar rationale, in Engelhardt's view, seems to motivate the focus on human ability, to take another of the medical values highlighted by him. Again the suggestion here is that physical (and mental changes) which impede human ability are devalued, and thus that maintenance of ability has a key place in medical approaches. So a person breaks an arm bone, thus disrupting their ability to play tennis. Restoration of the ability of the person to play tennis is a medical aim, since restoration of ability is valued and loss of ability devalued, according to Engelhardt. With regard to his reference to bodily form? The view seems to be that there are certain types of bodily form and of movement which are typical of humans and that the preservation of these, and restoration of them in cases of loss, constitute key medical goals. This is because Engelhardt sees deviation from certain species-typical morphology as an indication of pathology. It is because of this, I think, that 'ideal' bodily form is so important for Engelhardt's conception of medicine. Deviation is pathological in his view because of its association with the kinds of 'clusters of value judgements' previously discussed.

The idea of bodily form is also said by Engelhardt to raise aesthetic values ('deformity [is] ugly' (1996: 206). This rather extreme claim, symptomatic perhaps of an excessively constricted aesthetic sense, stems again in part from the close links Engelhardt sees between health and species-typical bodily form. If one locates these two, and is seduced into viewing them as co-extensive, then it will appear to follow that deviations from bodily form are devalued. I will return to this claim in a later discussion of aesthetic values.

Altogether then, medical values are manifested in acts which aim to relieve suffering, restore ability, including the ability to move in a species-typical way, and restore bodily form. These acts are driven by values relating to states of not suffering and the maintenance of bodily form and function.

There are two kinds of criticism which can be levelled at Engelhardt's point of view. The first is to reject the notion that medical values are of *intrinsic* significance as opposed to merely instrumental significance. To see this, consider the Alison Lapper statue mentioned above. She is a woman with an atypical bodily form. But it is implausible to think that this, in itself, would prompt medical interventions, for example to give her a typical bodily form. (This might be done, in the future, by some form of gene therapy.) The most likely reason why Alison Lapper's bodily form might be addressed is that if, as a consequence of her missing arms, her capacity to lead a full life is impugned. So if, because of her missing arms, she is unable to pursue a life plan that she would be happy with, then it may be that this would be a matter inviting consideration of some form of medical intervention. But the key consideration in assessing whether or not this is the case is not her bodily form in itself but the impact that bodily form has upon her capacity to pursue the kind of life she wishes.

The same applies to other medical values highlighted in Engelhardt's discussion. Suffering is only a medical matter if it impacts upon a person's capacity to pursue what they consider to be a good life. Some life plans may include endurance of suffering, and there the suffering is not a medical concern. These points show that Engelhardt's medical values are of instrumental rather than intrinsic significance. Relatedly, the discussion presented in this chapter also illustrates that valued states (being pain-free, being of a certain bodily form, being capable of a certain kind of bodily motion) connect up intimately with moral values. This is so because, for example, the significance of atypical bodily form depends upon its effects on a person's capacity to pursue the kind of life he or she wants to lead. And this is a moral concern. The same can be said in relation to other aspects which Engelhardt points to, that of relief from suffering and bodily movement: these are not significant in their own right, but by virtue of their impact upon one's capacity to pursue the kind of projects and life one wishes. Having considered medical values, I will now continue with consideration of moral values, in particular the views of Harris and then Nordenfelt.

Moral values

John Harris's claims, as previously mentioned, refer to moral values, in contrast to non-moral, medical ones. Moral values are those which drive many of our actions, especially when we try to 'do good' or to benefit others or to 'act fairly'. Harris apparently views disability as a harmed condition, one 'we have a strong rational preference not to be in' (2000: 97). This view involves moral values because such values lie behind precepts such as 'it is wrong to cause harm to others'. So to be in a harmed condition is to be in a negatively valued state. Note that it follows from such an account that there is a necessary relationship between having an impairment/disability and being in a devalued state. In other words, being disabled is an intrinsically negative state, a state preferably to be avoided. If one accepts this, it then follows that interventions such as prenatal screening programmes will seem justified. This is because every time the birth of a impaired/disabled child is prevented, a harm is prevented as well, if one accepts that disability is inevitably a harmed condition.

Why might one believe that impairment/disability is inevitably a harmed condition? Harris's answer to this question is that impairment causes 'the deprivation of worthwhile experience' (ibid.: 98). One can see that this claim has some (at least initial) plausibility, especially with regard to sensory impairments. If one is unable to hear one's child sing or laugh, or unable to see their face, then it can seem plausible to claim that in these circumstances the person is deprived of a range of worthwhile experiences.

Looking critically at Harris's views, it could be said that his account does not do sufficient justice to the actual experiences of people with sensory disabilities (see Vehmas 2004). Many might offer counter-arguments that there are experiences open only to them which are worthwhile, and so the deprivation of one class of experiences is offset, to some degree, by access to another class. Also, can it be coherent to claim that a person who is congenitally deaf or blind, say, is deprived of worthwhile experience if they have no conception of that kind of experience? Arguably, if they have never seen or heard, they may have no conception of what it is to see or to hear. In defence of Harris on this specific point though, he is open by pointing to situations in which it does seem coherent to say a person is deprived of something (x), even though they have never been in possession of (x); for example, one might say of children in a very poor country and in which there are no educational facilities, that they are deprived of education. This is a situation where it does seem coherent to say a person is deprived of something, although that something has never been previously had or experienced.

More problematically, how does Harris's conception of disability apply to people with a moderate intellectual disability and no accompanying sensory disabilities, in other words, a situation without an obvious set of sensory experiences of which the person is deprived? If pressed to think of a range of experiences where an intellectually disabled person might not have access, perhaps an example might be that he or she is incapable of processing complex cognitive tasks. But of course 'complexity' is a relative concept: what is complex for some is not so for others. For a mathematician, quadratic equations may be simple, whereas for a non-mathematician, they seem complex. For a young child, tying shoelaces can be a complex task. For an adult, typically it is not seen as complex. So, given the apparent relativity in the concept of complexity, this is not a promising strategy to save Harris's definition.

Moreover, it can appear extremely over-inclusive in the following way: compared to a musician with a finely tuned musical ear, my own sense of musical appreciation would be incredibly crude and blunt. Thus, I am deprived of that range of worthwhile experiences. Compared to the *gastronome*, my taste is similarly blunt and crude: insensitive to the subtleties in distinction available to him or her. Again, it seems I am deprived of a range of worthwhile experiences. The kinds of responses which are being made here could surely be made in relation to a very wide range of areas where worthwhile experiences are available to a specialist or expert, but not to the non-expert. It would seem to follow that we are all impaired/disabled, if Harris's definition is acceptable. His account might then be rejected on grounds of what might be termed 'over-inclusiveness'. This is because it seems plausible to think that a definition of disability should show us how to distinguish those that match its definitive characteristics from those that do not. But if a theory includes everyone, this is not possible, so the whole point of providing a definition in the first place goes missing.[2]

Also, what is lost in such an account is clarification of exactly what it is that would let us classify an experience as worthwhile. This seems a serious shortcoming, since it begs the question of how one distinguishes 'worthwhile' from other kinds of experiences. We need to know just what it is that makes us think of an experience as a worthwhile one. I think that judgements of that kind (regarding what is worthwhile as opposed to other types of experiences) are made against a background conception of what makes a 'good human life'. This is an illustration of the way in which discussions about disability presuppose some fairly deep ethical issues regarding what the components and conditions of a good human life might be. By 'a good human life', I do not necessarily mean 'a life doing good', but rather a life which would be a good one to lead: a fulfilling life. Ask what kind of life one would want for one's children. This then typically provides clues about what one believes to constitute a good life. According to Harris's line of argument, it appears as if having an impairment/disability either impugns one's capacity to lead a good life, or alternatively, makes it impossible to lead a good life. This view does not do justice to the value-orientations of disabled people themselves.

I will now move on to another perspective, that of Nordenfelt.

Nordenfelt

As mentioned in the introduction to this chapter, Nordenfelt has stated: 'The very classification of a person as handicapped presupposes an ethical or political decision' (2000: 123). This claim exemplifies again the place of values in discussions of disablement, in particular ethical values. The reference to political decisions in the above quote is simply to emphasise that such decisions inevitably have an ethical aspect. This is the case since all such decisions have some effect, beneficial or otherwise, on those on the receiving end of decisions.

Why does Nordenfelt take classifications of people as handicapped as stemming from an underlying ethical component? To appreciate this, it is necessary to briefly consider his definitions of disability and handicap. These comprise a crucial aspect of his general theory of disability, which in turn, is a component in his theory of health (Nordenfelt 1995, 2000).

Simply summarised, Nordenfelt considers a person to be disabled when one is unable to do things which are important to one. This inability must stem from a combination of internal factors (such as impairments) and external factors (such as wheelchair-unfriendly public transportation systems). He writes:

> A is handicapped with respect to action H, if and only if: H is a generated action. A is unable to perform H, given a specified set of circumstances that have been agreed upon in the context. A's performance of H is a necessary condition for the realisation of one or more of A's vital goals.
>
> (Nordenfelt 1993: 23)

It is not necessary to go into all the technical details of his account here (for further discussions, see Nordenfelt's other writings; and Edwards 2005). But, as mentioned, for Nordenfelt, one is handicapped when one is unable to pursue the things that are important to one, and when this stems from a combination of internal factors (e.g. the presence of an impairment) and external factors of the kind mentioned above. 'Vital goals' is the term which Nordenfelt deploys to signal the kinds of things which are important to a person's long-term well-being. Consider the following example: someone is unable to walk due to paraplegia, but bird-watching is very important, in fact so important that leading a good life is unthinkable without being able to pursue that activity. If one can pursue this interest and activity, say, by driving (or being driven) to the relevant places, and perhaps getting in and out of the car, then one is not handicapped according to Nordenfelt's definition. For one can pursue all those things which are important to one. (Assume for the sake of argument that this is the case.)

But now consider another person, Jim, who has severe intellectual disabilities. Suppose further that what Jim enjoys above everything else is watching films at the cinema. This is so important to Jim that it is credibly regarded as one of his vital goals. Suppose that hitherto, Jim has been supplied with a key support worker who takes him to the cinema on a daily basis. By Nordenfelt's definition, Jim is not handicapped. This is because he can fulfil his vital goals. (Again, for the sake of argument assume this is the case.)

Now suppose that a change in government policy in relation to social service expenditure occurs. Jim's key support worker is withdrawn. Visits to the cinema are no longer possible, Jim is too disabled to go alone, and there are insufficient numbers of support staff at Jim's residence to take him. Jim is now handicapped because he cannot pursue his vital goals. This illustrates Nordenfelt's point that the definition of a person as handicapped presupposes a political, and thereby an ethical, decision.

This discussion also illustrates again the intimate connection between impairment/disablement and values. Here a key dimension of disability/handicap, according to Nordenfelt, is shown to be inseparable from ethical decisions, which in turn embody ethical values. Furthermore, the more general ethical idea concerning what constitutes a good life for a person again comes to the forefront. At least as far as Jim is concerned, a good life is one which involves daily trips to the cinema. Nordenfelt's approach is important in assigning quite considerable weight to the values of the affected persons themselves. So again, it is evident that disablement and its dimensions have a core value component.

Having now presented this somewhat sympathetic illustration for the rationale behind Nordenfelt's view, I would like to highlight a couple of criticisms before moving on to looking at some other definitions. A first criticism of Nordenfelt's approach is that it may run the risk of subverting attempts at policy-making in relation to social provision for disabled people. This is because the conception of disability becomes personalised to such an extent that it could not be known whether or not people are disabled without actually asking them whether or not they (feel they) are able to achieve their vital goals. Some critics of Nordenfelt thus query the credibility of his notions on those grounds. Also, one might ask if it is possible to ameliorate all disabilities in the ways ameliorated in the two examples mentioned above (the bird-watcher and Jim). What about a person with such severe impairments/disabilities that they cannot conceive of, or express, any vital goals? If one meets their basic needs, for example, if their basic vital goals are for food, water, shelter, etc., surely they would still be impaired/disabled or 'handicapped'? There seems to be a range of problematic aspects in accepting Nordenfelt's approach, even though it appears plausible in relation to considering the lives of some people who would count as disabled according to other definitions (see Edward 1997; Nordenfelt 1999; Schramme 2007).

Other definitions

Readers will be aware of other definitions of disability besides those mentioned so far.

An early effort is the World Health Organisation's (WHO) *International Classification of Impairments, Disabilities and Handicaps (ICIDH)* (1980). Here the phenomenon of disablement is divided into three components: impairments, disabilities and handicaps, a way of thinking that has been much described and criticised (see Nordenfelt 1983, 1997; Oliver 1990; Edwards 2005). The purpose here is to draw attention to the value components contained within this definition.

A focus on the definition of impairment can help to illustrate the way in which values pervade even that, the most biological category. The definition of impairment includes reference to 'loss or abnormality of psychological, physiological or anatomical structure or function' (*ICIDH:* 27). It needs to be asked why a loss or an abnormality is of any significance, and once one begins to try to answer that question, one is inevitably drawn into the sphere of values. These might be aesthetic values relating to appearances judged to be displeasing or 'ugly' (Engelhardt 1996: 206). Or, they may also be moral values concerning the importance of specific kinds of lifestyle, such as being independent as opposed to dependent on others: if an impairment leads to a high level of dependency, it may become negatively valued because of this dependency-relationship. This is especially likely in contexts where great weight is attached to the notion of being an autonomous agent, where a centrally valued notion is that the autonomous agent is independent, not dependent upon others.

More prosaically, it might even be contended that terms such as 'loss' and 'abnormality' are in themselves value-laden. This certainly seems true of the term 'loss', as this is something typically disapproved of (although there are exceptions since 'loss' may be positively valued as in the loss of a cancerous tumour). At the very least, the term 'loss' is within the domain of value-stating discourse associated with negatively valued events.

With regard to the term 'abnormality', it is important to make a distinction between 'statistical descriptive' and 'normative' senses of 'abnormality' (Nordenfelt 1993: 18). The latter sense is employed in statements such as 'that is not normal', for example when expressing disapproval of a way of acting. Of course the statistical-descriptive and normative understandings can coincide, for example, when a kind of action is both rare and also disapproved of.

Additionally, in definitions regarding phenomena such as functions of organs, as the ICIDH does, the kinds of values which Engelhardt thinks of as non-moral, but rather as medical features. Parallel points can be made in relation to the more recent taxonomy provided by the WHO (ICF 2001). Although the category of 'impairments' is retained, the dimensions of disability and handicap are replaced by the terms 'activity limitations', and 'participation restrictions':

> Activity limitations are difficulties an individual may have in executing activities. An activity limitation may range from a slight to a severe deviation

in terms of quality or quantity in executing the activity in a manner or to the extent that is expected of people without the health condition.

(WHO, ICF 2001: 191)

The more social dimension of disablement is represented by the term 'participation restriction', defined as follows:

Participation restrictions are problems an individual may experience in involvement in life situations. The presence of a participation restriction is determined by comparing an individual's participation to that which is expected of an individual without disability in that culture or society.

(ibid.: 191)

A value component remains in this revised schema due to the retention of the concept of impairment. But the other two dimensions – activity limitations, and participation restrictions – seem again evaluative as the implication is that a limitation is undesirable, something to be addressed, as is a 'restriction'.

A definition of disability which preceded even the earlier WHO document is provided by the UPIAS (Union of the Physically Impaired Against Segregation), a definition considered a landmark in the development of the disability-rights movement in the UK. It marks a vivid assertion of the primacy of the perspective of disabled people themselves in disability issues, not least the very way in which disability is to be understood (see UPIAS 1975; Oliver 1990; Shakespeare 2006). It also asserts a forceful claim for an end to the exclusion of disabled people from social roles other than that of victim of a tragic event or patient (Oliver 1990).

As might be anticipated, the UPIAS definition is overtly value-laden, with its references to limbs labelled 'defective' and to phenomena such as exclusion and restrictions. Consider the following definitions:

Impairment: lacking part or all of a limb, or having a defective limb, organ or mechanism of the body.
Disability: the disadvantage or restriction of activity caused by a contemporary social organisation which takes little or no account of people who have physical impairments and thus excludes them from participation in the mainstream of social activities.

(quoted in Oliver 1990: 11; UPIAS 1975)

Moreover, the UPIAS definition 'locates the causes of disability squarely within society and social organisation' (Oliver 1990: 11). As pointed out in the previous discussion of Nordenfelt's definition, political decisions can affect categories such as 'disabled' and 'non-disabled' depending upon ethical values and upon how disability is defined. But the UPIAS definition, in emphasising the social element of the causation of disability, runs the risk of neglecting the biological element to disability (Shakespeare 2006). Nor is it clear how sensory and intellectual disabilities are encompassed.

As thus far argued, a considerable range of definitions of disability presuppose some value elements. These may be medical ones concerning function and form, or moral values relating to what is harmful, or normal in an evaluative sense. I have also tried to indicate that at a deeper level, definitions of disability presuppose some underlying value concerning what is a good life for a human being (this idea is developed in more detail in Edwards 2005; Vehmas 2004).

In the final section, I return to discuss the last quote presented in the introduction to this chapter. This is from the artist Alison Lapper and involves aesthetic values. I will then also revisit Engelhardt's remarks concerning deformity.

Aesthetic values

What about aesthetic values and disability issues? This question is particularly prompted by the statue of Alison Lapper. The statue is a representation of her naked, pregnant and lacking arms. It was produced by sculptor Marc Quinn and caused some controversy when first displayed in public in Trafalgar Square, London on 15 September 2005.

Reactions to the statue were varied, as might perhaps be expected. Some regarded it very positively (including the model herself) and others were unhappy about the statue for a range of reasons. There may be some connection between the kind of views expressed in Engelhardt's remarks about the 'ugliness' of deformity and some of the negative responses to the statue. For the sake of discussion, let us understand the term 'deformity' as a deviation from species-typical morphology. Alison Lapper's body is 'deformed' in that sense since it is species-typical for humans to have two arms of a certain length. She lacks these and so counts as deformed according to that way of defining deformity.

The relevant type of values in play here with regard to judgements about the statue and about deformity (to persist with Engelhardt's term) are aesthetic values. These are manifested in judgements which invoke conceptions such as beauty and ugliness. So, for example, works of art paradigmatically instantiate aesthetic properties. Critics then advance aesthetic judgements concerning the merits (or lack thereof) of the works of art. In the context of disability, aesthetic values have been discussed in the past concerning people with Down Syndrome who have had plastic surgery to alter their appearance in such a way that it is not evident from looking at them that they have that syndrome (Edwards 1996).

The position captured in Engelhardt's claim is helpful in a way, because it is such a strong and extreme claim: that there is a necessary connection between deformity and negatively valued aesthetic properties. In other words, that the aesthetic values prompted by the sight of deformity will inevitably be negative. The mixed reaction to the statue shows that this is not the case. Yet, how might Engelhardt respond in defence of his claim? One option would be to argue that those for whom the statue provokes negative aesthetic value judgements ('that's ugly', 'that's repulsive', etc.) are correct. Their aesthetic sense is correctly 'tuned' so to speak. The others are simply mistaken.

But how plausible is this? Aesthetic properties do not seem to be the kind of properties about which it is possible to be certain that one judgement is correct and another incorrect. That is one explanation for the disagreements which beset the art world, where critics cannot agree on the merits of a specific work of art. Some kinds of judgements, are about simple matters of fact ('there are two chairs in this room'), with little scope for genuine dispute. But in aesthetic matters this is not so. So, the strong claim advanced by Engelhardt is, I would argue, almost certainly false. And the Lapper statue, and the mixed responses it has provoked, lend some support to my view. In addition, again in opposition to Engelhardt's strong claim, it is well documented that changes in matters of aesthetic taste vary across cultures and across historical periods. It is not clear that there is one common aesthetically ideal human form which is universally positively valued. So the idea that deformity is intrinsically negatively valued does not seem promising. And even if a person is initially disturbed by the sight of a person with a radically abnormal appearance, continued interaction with that person typically reduces the initial negative aesthetic evaluation. If deformity were intrinsically ugly, this would not happen. So Engelhardt's strong claim need not be accepted.

Concluding comments

I began by presenting the views of four commentators relating to disability, suggesting that each view incorporates some claim(s) about value. These were then said to be, respectively medical, moral, and aesthetic. I have used that lens to review some common definitions of disability and to try to expose their evaluative element. What is more difficult is to try to demonstrate that one person's opinion about a value-impregnated matter is accurate and another is definitely false. This is well illustrated in the discussion of aesthetic values. In the discussions of moral and medical values, as was the case in the discussion of aesthetic values, hopefully, it has been evident that there seem good reasons for giving great weight to the opinions of disabled people themselves in relation to definitional matters. As mentioned, although these can never be indisputable, there are good moral grounds to assign them more weight. Such a position falls between an 'objectivist line' according to which there is an objectively discoverable state which constitutes being disabled, and a 'subjectivist' line according to which the question of whether or not a person is disabled is determined entirely by their own opinion (Vehmas 2004). The line of argument presented in this chapter is that the views of people who regard themselves as disabled in some sense, should be accorded due weight.

Notes

1 See also Vehmas (2004: 214): 'the essential core of the concept of disability is ethical.'
2 This inclusiveness could be a strength of Harris's definition – see the idea of 'universalism' in the WHO's ICF (2001). According to this, disability is indeed a universal experience, one to be anticipated by all humans at some stage in their lives. This is brought out in Bickenbach's explication of the ICF when he writes, 'Disablement

'... is an intrinsic feature of the human condition, not a difference that essentially marks one sub-population off from another' (Bickenbach *et al.* 1999: 17).

Bibliography

Bickenbach, J. E., Chatterji, S., Badley, E. M. and Ustun, T. B. (1999) 'Models of Disablement, Universalism and the ICIDH', *Social Science and Medicine*, 48: 1173–87.

Edwards, S. D. (1996) 'Plastic Surgery and Individuals with Down's Syndrome', in I. de Beaufort, S. Holm and M. Hilhorst (eds), *The Eye of the Beholder: Ethics and Medical Change of Appearance*, Oslo: Scandinavian University Press.

—— (2005) *Disability, Definition, Value and Identity*, Oxford: Radcliffe Press.

Engelhardt, T. (1996) *The Foundations of Bioethics*, Oxford: Oxford University Press.

Harris, J. (2000) 'Is There a Coherent Social Conception of Disability?', *Journal of Medical Ethics*, 26: 95–100.

Nordenfelt, L. (1983) *On Disabilities and their Classification*, Linköping: University of Linköping Press.

—— (1993) 'On the Notions of Disability and Handicap', *Social Welfare*, 2: 17–24.

—— (1995) *On the Nature of Health*, Dordrecht: Kluwer.

—— (1999) 'On Disability and Illness: A Reply to Edwards', *Theoretical Medicine*, 20: 181–9.

—— (2000) *Action, Ability and Health*, Dordrecht: Kluwer.

Oliver, M. (1990) *The Politics of Disablement*, London: Macmillan.

Ouch! (2005) 'Alison Lapper Pregnant Unveiled', available online at < http://www.bbc.co.uk/print/ouch/news/btn/lapper/index.shtml > (accessed 16 November 2006).

Schramme, T. (2007) 'A Qualified Defence of a Naturalist Theory of Health', *Medicine, Health Care and Philosophy*, 10: 11–17.

Shakespeare, T. (2007) *Disability Rights and Wrongs*, London and New York: Routledge.

Union of the Physically Impaired against Segregation (UPIAS) (1975) *Fundamental Principles of Disability*, London: UPIAS.

Vehmas, S. (2004) 'Ethical Analysis of the Concept of Disability', *Mental Retardation*, 42: 209–22.

World Health Organisation (WHO) (1980) *International Classification of Impairments, Disabilities and Handicaps*, Geneva: WHO.

—— (2001) *International Classification of Functioning, Disability and Health*, Geneva: WHO.

3 The ontology of disability and impairment

A discussion of the natural and social features

Simo Vehmas and Pekka Mäkelä

Introduction

Nowadays it is widely acknowledged that disability is not merely a matter of biological impairment but also, and perhaps primarily, a social phenomenon; disablement cannot be explained and understood simply in terms of people's impairment
but, rather, in terms of social arrangements. In other words, it is not individuals and their alleged incapacities that explain the limited opportunities of people
with impairments; society is partly to blame as well. This sociological perspective
typically represented and promoted in the increasingly popular field of disability
studies rejects essentialistic views of human beings. What is considered as characteristically 'human' or 'normal' with regard to the make-up of beings does not
depend on human essence (whatever that might be), but on culturally produced
norms. Humanity and normality are socially constructed. Social constructionism
can thus be seen as the ontological and epistemological basis of disability studies,
and consequently it has become the framework for understanding what disability
is all about, as well as how one construes information about it (Albrecht 2002;
Barnes *et al.* 1999: 93–5; Linton 1998: 37–45; Taylor 1996).[1]

Briefly, the social constructionist view of disability tends to contend that:

1. Disability is not the same as impairment, and cannot be understood properly
    on the basis of impairment. Although the notion of equating impairment with
    disability is deeply rooted in our culture, it is not determined by the nature of
    things; it is not inevitable.
2. The 'Western' conception of disability as an individual's biological condition
    is incorrect and harmful.
3. We would be much better off if the individualistic way of thinking concern-
    ing disability were done away with, or at least radically transformed (see
    Hacking 1999: 6).

There are various differing accounts of what disability as a social construct means
in practice. One constant complication in these discussions is the role, meaning
and significance of body and impairment. This problem concerns especially the
(largely British) materialist research tradition (i.e., the social model of disability)

which defines disability as a form of social oppression and hence as a phenomenon that should be conceptualised in social terms. Consistently, individual properties, such as impairments, are not regarded as crucial in this approach which has focused on analysing the social causes of disability. In Britain the study of impairment was soon pushed to the fringes of disability studies (e.g., Hughes 2002; Thomas 2002). Many have argued that this has been a serious shortcoming in the social model of disability, arguing instead that any theoretical account attempting to explain and theorise disability satisfactorily needs to take into account corporeal issues (e.g., Shakespeare 2006; Morris 1991; Thomas 1999; Wendell 1996; Williams 1999; see also Scully in this book). However, as opposed to the strict materialist view, many scholars define disability in terms of functional limitations, and in doing so, they are forced to acknowledge the significance of impairments (Hughes 2002; Shakespeare and Watson 2001; Thomas 1999: 40–2; 2004a, 2004b).

Altogether, one of the most constant and pressing issues in the social-constructionist tradition of disability studies is the meaning of impairment. To what extent are bodily features intrinsic properties and to what extent social constructs? Accordingly, in addition to the sociology of disability, there is a growing amount of literature on the sociology of impairment. The enterprise of constructing a sociology of impairment has largely been a reaction and antithesis to accounts labelled as modernist. The traditional medical view of disability, as well as the British social model of disability, have been accused as treating the body 'as a pre-social, inert, physical object, as discrete, palpable and separate from the self' (Hughes and Paterson 1997: 329). Both of these accounts are seen to be inaccurate because of presenting a one-sided view of impairments and bodies as biological entities: 'the impaired body has a history and is as much a cultural phenomenon as it is a biological entity' (Paterson and Hughes 1999: 600).

The postmodern crusade for and against the corpus

The discussions about the sociology of impairment have, to a considerable extent, evolved around theorising in realms that are typically termed postmodern or poststructuralist. What unites this diverse criticism levelled at theories cursed with Cartesian leanings is their dismissal of dualistic explanations. A Cartesian worldview has produced a number of dichotomies where, for example, human beings are seen to be constituted of two separate entities, namely mind and body. For instance, the social model of disability has been accused of falling into a modernistic trap where disability is seen as social and political, and impairment as biological and personal. Many postmodernist scholars have compellingly argued that things are not that simple. Entities considered as purely physical or biological, such as impairments, are also cultural and social entities (Hughes 1999; Morris 1991; Shakespeare 2006; Shakespeare and Watson 2001; Thomas 1999; Wendell 1996).

We have no quarrel whatsoever with positions building on the basic idea of disability as a social category and social construction. We also have no problem acknowledging that impairments are both biological and cultural entities. It should be noted at this point that in our terminology *impairment* is a class name for natural properties that, depending on the context, in part cause or constitute functional limitations – although the limiting implications of the property in question can in part be explained in social terms. Impairment always involves a physical element, a condition of some sort which is seen as undesirable regarding people's organic or social functioning. Thus, impairment is a physical or organic phenomenon whose identification and definition are determined culturally and socially; it is inevitably about attaching some meaning to individual properties. *Disability*, however, is a relational phenomenon that consists in the relation between the natural properties or features on the one hand, and the surrounding social and physical world on the other. Disability is in its nature and is inevitably, and self-evidently, a social construct. What distinguishes disability from impairment is that it can become dissociated from people's physical conditions. Disability often involves very general social structures and mechanisms that cannot be reduced to people's physical or mental characteristics. Disability has started to have a life of its own, as it were. Thus, disability as a social phenomenon does not necessarily require impairment in the proper sense; some individual features and ways of acting can become labelled as impairments although they may have no verifiable organic basis.

Despite our naturalist inclinations, we think that our account in this chapter about the ontology of disability and impairment is to a large extent a reconciling view between the extreme medical and extreme social positions. Also, at its core, our contribution is actually (social) constructionist because it aims at 'displaying or analyzing actual, historically situated, social interactions or causal routes that led to, or were involved in, the coming into being or establishing of some present entity or fact' (Hacking 1999: 48).

So, in our view there is nothing radical at all in conceptualising disability in terms of constructionism. However, some points that certain disability scholars have stated about impairment on the basis of postmodern ideas, and the entailments thereof, appear to us as peculiar, confusing and even unhelpful. What is one to make of statements such as the following: 'impairment and its materiality are naturalised *effects* of disciplinary knowledge/power' (Tremain 2002: 34)? Does this mean that impairments are not primarily or even secondarily biological facts but historically contingent effects of power based on professional expertise and knowledge? In addition, is the following extract suggesting that intellectual impairments, for instance, do not have a biological grounding prior to representation: 'without the *prior* existence of language, such "psychological" things as "intellectual (dis)abilities", "syndromes" … can, quite literally, not sensibly be talked of' (Goodley and Rapley 2002: 128).[2] In other words, are impairments not matters of physical entity, but rather of representation, discourse and social construction? Should impairments as words be placed in apostrophes? 'Impairment in the modern, materialist world remains characteristically biological and not an aspect of disabled people's lives that can or should be changed' (ibid. 2002: 133). Can and should the alleged impairment and possible incompetence related to, for example, Down syndrome be abolished merely by re- and deconstructing the impairment? Or are impairments merely allegories or myths for something completely different? 'It [mental retardation] is a reification – a socially created category which is assumed to have an existence independent of its creators' minds. ... Mental retardation is a misnomer, a myth' (Bogdan and Taylor 1994: 7). Whilst Bogdan and Taylor suggest that mental retardation should not be understood as an objective fact, they do not deny that there are differences among people in terms of intellectual ability but rather that the nature and significance of these differences depend on how we view and interpret them.

Numerous similar extracts can be found in the disability studies literature (e.g., Danforth 2000; Danforth and Rhodes 1997; Goodley 2001; Hughes 1999; Hughes and Paterson 1997; Roets *et al.* 2007; Shildrick and Price 1996) that leave philosophers with realist leanings, such as us, perplexed and confused. It seems to us that the common rhetoric in disability studies suggests an extreme form of social constructionism, or linguistic idealism (Hacking 1999: 24), which, when consistently applied, leads to the conclusion that impairments are not primarily or even secondarily biological facts; nothing exists until it is spoken of or written about. Impairments are represented as kinds of artefacts (see Best 2007). Such a relativist leaning that denies reality outside of discourse and text, is in-built in social-constructionist thinking, although many critical social constructionists oppose such a tendency (Burr 2003: 23). However, in disability studies there exists a linguistic attempt to challenge the reality of impairment. Phrases such as 'people who are viewed by others as having some form of impairment' (Oliver 2004: 21) and placing terms such as 'learning difficulties' in apostrophes (Goodley 2001), seem to suggest that these conditions do not have an objective organic basis (Shakespeare 2006: 39). This tendency is a consistent outcome of a postmodern train of thought, one which denies the possibility of recapturing or even representing the origin, source, or any deeper reality outside the phenomena, and casts doubt on, or even denies its existence: no natural givens precede the processes of social determination (Cahoone 2002: 15; Fuss 1989: 2–3).

Simon Williams has pointed out that despite their linguistic commitment to corporeal issues, the postmodernists totally diminish the body by reducing it to discourse and representation. As a result, what we have is a discursive body, 'one whose matter really doesn't matter at all' (Williams 1999: 804). Now, we do not wish to stake a claim for a monopoly of proper reading of the poststructuralist account of disability, but we do think that our interpretation is plausible, and the concerns raised here are reasonable. So, we think that the sociology of impairment discourse in disability studies lacks proper ontological scrutiny and basis. From our standpoint, the ontology of impairment needs to be resolved before one can understand and explain the phenomenon of disability satisfactorily.

In this chapter, we address some epistemological and ontological questions of impairment and disability. What is impairment all about? Is it just physical or just social, or something in between? What is its relationship to disablement? Can impairments be (socially) constructed? In our view, impairment includes both a physical and social dimension. We argue that impairments have a grounding in physical facts which is a necessary condition for any of the social functions of impairment. We are not under the illusion that we could provide an extensive account of the ontology of disability and impairment. However, we present a realist framework which hopefully avoids the pitfalls and obscurities of postmodern accounts and also offers a more plausible and clearer basis for our understanding of the phenomenon of disability.

Intrinsic and observer-relative features of the world

Do impairments exist intrinsically or should they be primarily understood as linguistic artefacts? A conceptual clarification is in order to resolve this dilemma. First, there is an important distinction between the senses of 'objective' and 'subjective' with regard to epistemology and ontology. Epistemic sense of objective–subjective distinction refers to discussions about our judgements of how things are in the world and their truth (or credibility). A judgement is subjective if its truth (or correctness) depends on the attitudes, feelings, or points of view of the maker and the hearer of the judgement. An example of such a judgement could be: 'Jane Austen is a better writer than Emily Brontë.' A judgement is objective if its truth is settled by facts in the world that are independent of the maker and hearer of the judgement. In other words, if a statement is objective in the epistemic sense, then there is an objective fact in the world which makes it true. Such a statement would be, for instance, 'Jane Austen was born on 1775 in Steventon, Hampshire.' The contrast between epistemic objectivity and epistemic subjectivity is a matter of degree (Searle 1995: 8).

In the ontological sense, objective and subjective are predicates of the entities in the world, types of entities and their mode of existence. Objective entities exist independently of any perceiver or mental state, whereas subjective entities are dependent on perceivers and mental states. So, in the ontological sense, pains are subjective entities because their existence depends on the subject's experience. But mountains, for example, are ontologically objective because their mode of existence is independent of any perceiver: mountains would remain in the world even if all the humans and other subjects with senses disappeared from the earth. Here we need to distinguish between the senses of objective and subjective, that is, we can make epistemically subjective statements about entities that are ontologically objective, and similarly, we can make epistemically objective statements about entities that are ontologically subjective. For example, the statement 'It is better not to have an extra chromosome 21 than to have it' is about an ontologically objective entity, but makes a subjective judgement about it. On the other hand, the statement 'The fact that my child has an extra chromosome 21 causes me emotional distress' reports an epistemically objective fact in the sense that it is made true by the existence of an actual fact that is not dependent on any opinion of observers. Nevertheless, the phenomenon itself, the actual emotional distress, has a subjective mode of existence (ibid.: 8–9).

Another crucial distinction related to the existence of things prior to representation is between *intrinsic* and *observer-relative* features of the world. Let us imagine, for example, an object that a person who has paralysed legs sits on and moves about with. The object has a certain mass and a certain chemical composition. It is made, for example, of metal, plastic and rubber, all of which are composed of certain molecules. All of these features are undoubtedly intrinsic. However, it is also true to say of the very same object that it is a wheelchair. When we name or describe it as a wheelchair, we are specifying a feature of the object that is observer or user-relative. It is a wheelchair only because people use it as a wheelchair. The mere concept of wheelchair implies a certain user-relative function and purpose of the object. The observer-relative features of the world do not add any material objects to reality, but they can add epistemically objective features to reality where the features in question exist relative to observers and users. In other words, it is an epistemically objective feature of this object that it is a wheelchair, but since that feature exists only relative to observers and users, the feature is ontologically subjective (ibid.: 9–10). John Searle sums up this thesis in the following way: 'Observer-relative features exist only relative to the attitudes of observers. Intrinsic features don't give a damn about observers and exist independently of observers' (ibid.: 11).

Impairments: brute facts or institutional facts?

Before the issue of impairments, syndromes and the like which exist prior to representation can be settled, a few more considerations concerning conceptual distinctions are required. Searle argues that there are features of the world that are matters of brute physics and biology and, on the other hand, features that are matters of culture and society. Although these two dimensions are related to each other, to some extent they can and should be separated. Brute facts, such as the fact that Mount Everest has snow and ice near the summit, are those that require no human institution for their existence, whereas institutional facts can exist only within human institutions, such as the fact that Joseph Ratzinger is Benedict XVI, the current Pope of the Catholic Church. To state a brute fact of course requires the institution of language, but the fact stated is not the same as the statement of it (Searle 1995: 27). Thus, the *statement* that someone has appendicitis requires an institution of language and an institution (i.e., medicine) of identifying organic functions and their outcomes, but the *fact stated*, the fact that someone's appendix becomes infected, exists independently of language or any other institution.

Brute facts do not require language or representation for their existence, whereas institutional facts do. One obvious example of a class of such facts is *declarations*, speech acts in which 'the state of affairs represented by the propositional content of the speech act is brought into existence by the successful performance of that very speech act' (ibid.: 34). Institutional facts can thus be created with the performative utterance of such sentences as 'I now pronounce you husband and wife' or 'War is hereby declared'. An example of such a performative utterance in the disability context would be that of diagnosis: someone's impairment starts to exist institutionally when a doctor proclaims a diagnosis. In the case of most institutional facts, the linguistic element appears to be partly constitutive of the fact. We could not have presidents, queens, husbands, wives or, let alone, disabled people, unless we had the apparatus necessary to represent some people as, for example, presidents or disabled (ibid.: 37).

But before we can name or agree upon any facts, that is, to have institutional facts, we have to have brute facts. In order to have money, games, schools, medical diagnoses or any other human institution, there must be some physical realisation, some brute fact on which we can impose a social function. All sorts of substances can be money. Whether it is bits of metal, pieces of paper, magnetic traces on plastic cards, it has to exist in some physical form. More generally, social facts, and institutional facts in particular, are hierarchically structured. Institutional facts exist on top of brute facts, as it were. Brute facts, for their part, do not have to be restricted to physical objects: sounds, marks on paper, or even thoughts in people's heads can count as brute facts (see ibid.: 34–5).

Thus, the brute level of facts is the necessary foundation of institutional facts. However, institutional facts cannot exist without social conventions and without representation (ibid.: 68). Social phenomena inevitably have a social history. Hughes and Paterson, for instance, are quite right for criticising accounts that construct body and impairment purely in biological terms (Hughes and Paterson 1997). But this does not mean that impairment is primarily, or let alone wholly socially produced. The diagnosis of trisomy 21 (or Down syndrome) has a social history, one with various social consequences for the lives of those with that diagnosis. However, despite the fact that trisomy 21 is a construction, an invented term for a certain phenomenon, it is also a term for an existing physical fact. Irrespective of any construction or representation, someone either has or does not have an extra chromosome 21. The existence of an extra chromosome 21 does not have a social history, it merely has a mere biological history. In other words, the diagnosis 'Down syndrome' is not a sole creation of anatomy and physiology, whereas the existence of an extra chromosome 21 is.

On a purely organic level, the existence of a certain chromosome is not in any way dependent upon representation. But the naming of this particular biological phenomenon as an *extra* chromosome 21 shifts us from a brute level to an institutional level. This is because defining some entity as 'extra' implies that it is seen vis-à-vis biological laws or statistics and the way organisms of this kind usually are.[3] Most of all, however, the definition of this syndrome (as with all other syndromes) is related to the functions ascribed to organs and organisms. For example, we are aware of certain causal processes in human bodies having to do with survival of the organism. When we say 'The heart pumps blood' we are recording an intrinsic, brute fact. But when we say 'The function of the heart is to pump blood', we are situating this intrinsic fact into a system of values that we hold. When we assign a function to something, it means that to us this substance has a task to fulfil or is a means to something: 'Functions, in short, are never intrinsic but are always observer relative' (Searle 1995: 14). When we have assigned a function to the heart or any other organ, we can use the vocabulary of success in relation to them, that is, we can speak of malfunction, or better and worse hearts. We could not do this if we talked about simple brute facts of nature.

The condition named extra chromosome 21 or Down syndrome, includes a brute fact of nature. However, it also includes an institutional level, not just epistemically (which is always linked to representation) but also ontologically. This is because this condition is very much related to the values and purposes that we have assigned to different organs (as in relation to the purposes of human bodies and minds). An extra chromosome 21 is an example of a brute fact that is identified and understood in relation to a system of values. It has been recognised that this brute fact is statistically correlated with certain biological features. But this brute fact implies some social consequences as well. In fact, Down syndrome is very much a social category. The need to define and identify this condition in newborn babies and foetuses is based on social expectations that can be seen as twofold: (1) expectations of how human beings ought to develop and what kinds of beings they should develop into; and (2) expectations that individuals with Down syndrome are unlikely to develop in ways deemed desirable.

Additionally, recognising an extra chromosome 21 in some individuals has major social consequences for their lives (or in other words, identifying brute facts may have major institutional outcomes for people). The crucial outcome is that these individuals will be seen by most people primarily in relation to their organic condition. We have developed various institutions for these people: we have highly advanced techniques to detect this brute fact in individuals during pregnancy in order to prevent their birth (in fact, preventing the birth of such children has turned into a massive endeavour and an institution of its own in Western medical practice). We have also constructed establishments specifically for children with these kinds of conditions to rear and educate them. We have various procedures to prevent them from reproducing (in the case their biological condition does not prevent it), from participating in social and professional life, and so on and so forth (Baron *et al.* 1998; Barton 1998; Vehmas 2003). In other words, the brute fact of a body often determines an individual's institutional life in a way that can be depicted as brutal.

The construction of 'social impairments'

The ontology of impairments whose etiology is known and certain seems quite straightforward: the organic entities, such as extra chromosome 21, are brute physical facts, whereas our knowledge of those facts and their impact on people's lives is always at least partly socially constructed. However, things are more complicated in the case of those people who are seen to have significant problems in their behavioural and social lives. In other words, what are we to make of diagnoses such as Attention Deficit Hyperactivity Disorder (ADHD) or Asperger's syndrome, to what extent are they brute or institutional facts? Is there in any meaningful sense such things as *social* impairments? Can 'bad' or 'mad' behaviour be depicted as a brute fact?

Psychiatric conditions in general are classified on symptomatic grounds (Hacking 1995: 12). Often scientists have not been able to verify a particular organic cause for a certain characteristic or behaviour. Rather, diagnoses are based on observations about certain people's problematic characteristics and behaviour. When certain behaviours are identified or constructed, people who are exhibiting those behaviours are diagnosed or labelled as having schizophrenia, ADHD, Asperger's, and so on. All this seems to imply that, for example, habits named as 'behavioural disorders' are wholly language dependent because the corresponding facts are language dependent. There is no fact of the matter about the thought 'Today is Thursday the 9th of August' except the fact that it occupies a position relative to a verbal system. But isn't that also true of, for instance, dogs? Isn't something correctly called a 'dog' only relative to a linguistic system and a system for identifying animals? No, because 'the features in virtue of which it is a dog, are features that exist independently of language' (Searle 1995: 65). The same applies to conditions such as trisomy 21 and spina bifida because they are clearly verifiable brute facts.

However, intellectual disability, behavioural disorder or any other categorisation of human beings cannot be a brute fact because social and institutional facts are not 'out there' in the way that planets, dogs, chromosomes or neural tubes are (see ibid.: 68). Similarly, assault is not 'out there' whereas a punch in the nose is most certainly 'out there'. The same applies to all human encounters, relationships and behaviours: something does happen physically but exactly *what* happens is determined institutionally.

Neuropsychiatric diagnoses can be seen to be parallel with speech acts that create institutional facts, such as marriage, which in turn create status-functions, namely, that of husband and wife. These status functions carry specific rights and obligations that were imposed on people by the speech acts performed, in this case in a marriage ceremony (ibid.: 83). Diagnosing someone with, for example, ADHD creates an institutional fact but not as clearly a status function with consequent rights and obligations in the same way as pronouncing a couple as husband and wife does. What psychiatric diagnosis may very well produce is, in the words of Ian Hacking (1995), the *looping effect* of human kinds. The looping effect refers to the process where 'people classified in a certain way tend to conform to or grow into the ways that they are described; but they also evolve in their own ways, so that the classifications and descriptions have to be constantly revised' (ibid.: 21). Diagnoses and people with those diagnoses are thus 'moving targets because our investigations interact with the targets themselves, and change them. And since they are changed, they are not quite the same kind of people as before. The target has moved' (ibid.: 2). New classifications of people or of behaviour may create new ways to be a person, new choices to be made, and, because of this, new opportunities for action are opened to these people. Previously, certain people were described as introverted, obsessive and asocial or impulsive and energetic. Now they are described as having Asperger's or ADHD with the result that new ways to be introverted, obsessive and asocial as well as new ways to be impulsive and energetic have been created, as well (see Hacking 1995: 236, 239).

Thus, diagnoses can, in a sense, be described with the slogan 'making up people' (Hacking 2006: 2), where the new (scientific) descriptions of people change their sense of self-worth and reorganise and re-evaluate their identity. It has been argued that in practice defining people's behaviour as a biological and a medical problem has, among other problems, passivised, not empowered people labelled as having, for example, ADHD or Asperger's because their supposed problems are out of their control (e.g., Cooper 2001; Levine 1997). Hence, they cannot be responsible for their actions, nor can the surrounding environment and institutions (e.g., schools) do much since deep down the cause of the problem is in the individual's physical properties. From this viewpoint, diagnosis works as a *status indicator* (see Searle 1995: 85) which demonstrates the 'patient's' position in relation to professionals (e.g., physicians) and institutions (e.g., schools). Thus, diagnoses as status-functions and status indicators create power positions (ibid.: 95–6). If A is a doctor who diagnoses B as having ADHD, A has power over B to intervene in B's life and body.

Thus, new diagnoses and classifications create new kinds of human beings and new kinds of relationships between people. For example, homosexual and hetero-sexual as kinds of persons came into being only towards the end of the nineteenth century. There has always been same-sex activity, but not same-sex people and different-sex people until the distinction was made (Hacking 1986: 225). Similarly, diagnoses such as ADHD have created for certain people new identities and new personalities and thus new ways to live socially. They also enable people to revise or even reinvent their personal narratives. With a new understanding about their personalities, people are able to give different meanings to past events and actions: they can rethink, redescribe, and refeel the past. In a sense, the past becomes filled with actions that were not there when they were performed (see Hacking 1995: 249–53). For example, a bad-mannered, wayward brat may turn into helpless child who could not know any better. He or she was simply a victim of a physical condition.

When the stories of our lives change, we change as well. With new descriptions we can call for new identities and personalities. And, 'the tighter the chain of causation – the more specific etiology – the better the narrative' (ibid.: 256). That is, in contemporary Western cultures dominated by the medical discourse, our new identity appears to rest on more solid ground when it has a credible scientific explanation: epicrisis has become the official biography of the deviant person. This general sympathy with the medico-scientific discourse may be one reason for the common urge to believe in simplistic neurological and materialistic explana-tions about people's characters and behaviour.

Ontology and disability politics

Debates about the true nature of disability are heated probably because of the close connection of ontology to politics. In the West, deviance has been under-stood either in terms of morality or medicine. In this case, impairment can be seen as result of people's moral flaws or of their pathological conditions (see Silvers 1998: 56–9). These kinds of views have had a great, and often a dreadful, impact on the lives of people with impairments. So, it is quite understandable that the fight concerning the epistemological dominance over disability is fierce. The one with the best story is supposedly seen to win the political battle as well.

One reason for the dominance of social constructionism in disability studies is its political usefulness. Talk of construction undermines the authority of knowledge and authorisation and thus provides legitimacy to the subjective voices of people with impairments. Social constructionism challenges naturalised truths considered as inevitable by unmasking these assumptions: 'The point of unmasking is to liberate the oppressed, to show how categories of knowledge are used in power relationships' (Hacking 1999: 58). In the case of many neuro-psychiatric diagnoses, the unmasking is undoubtedly necessary if the construction of a psychiatric identity compromises one's well-being and social status. And since problems in social behaviour and competence are necessarily dialogical phenomena that cannot possibly be understood merely in terms of an individual and his or her characteristics, the danger of discrimination is apparent in the categorisation of people on the basis of their psychological identities. This would seem to suggest that, for example, controlling people's behaviour by affecting their bodies with medication is a morally dubious endeavour.[4]

In some disability studies traditions, the talk about oppression has become a sort of unquestioned mantra – there seems to be no context where you could not accuse someone of oppressing disabled people, and the burden of proof is always on those who question this notion. One example of such tendency is the following quote by Goodley and Rapley (2002: 138) who claim that 'naturalised views of impairment are at the core of oppression'. These kinds of statements are consistent outcomes of the research tradition adopted among the British disability studies community where validity of research is measured by political standards and requires the adoption of a social model of disability as the ontological and epistemological basis for research production (Barnes 1996; Barnes and Sheldon 2007; Mercer 2002; Oliver 1992; Stone and Priestley 1996). It appears that in this 'emancipatory research' tradition, the requirement is to derive 'is' from 'ought'; that is, to have an ontology which best serves the aims and goals of the (possibly noble) political agenda (Vehmas 2008).

Our attempt in this chapter to understand the ontology and construction of the phenomena of impairment and disability is primarily descriptive, and from where we stand does not seem to involve any political or other normative commitments whatsoever. It does involve a methodological commitment to the idea that we should get our ontology right before we build agendas to change the status quo. This does not imply closing one's eyes to the moral and political issues involved in the subject matter. Quite the opposite, we tend to think that the fruitful discussion of moral and political issues is better served with the kind of ontological position defended here than with any extreme position that denies the relevance of the undeniable, constitutive parts of the phenomenon.

For example, if a person's certain physical property classified as impairment results in disabling and oppressive treatment in a certain social context, the first and the right thing to do would appear to be to change the social arrangements of the context, if possible. However, social structures, practices, arrangements, value structures and so on, are notoriously difficult and slow to change. This is quite understandable since they are collectively created and maintained, and also historically deep-rooted. This being the case, it may actually be more appropriate to change the physical property of the person itself *if* it is the only way to increase the well-being of that person during his or her lifetime. This is not to deny that the physical property developed its unfortunate implications with respect to the well-being of the individual due to the indecent attitudinal climate of the social context which, of course, is highly unacceptable.

Thus, recognising a state of affairs is not to accept the status quo. Therefore, recognising that a physical property may in some contexts lead to oppressive treatment of the owners of that property does not imply the acceptance of this situation. However, if the ontology discussed above unmasks and thus *constructs* the phenomena of disability and impairment along the right lines, then we have more tools in our tool-kit to try to change the state of affairs than we would have if we denied the relevance of the physical features of impairment and disability. An ontology that emphasises the physical origins of impairment and the relational nature of disability enables us to eradicate both organic and social factors that have resulted in people's distress. In other words, we can be more flexible and efficient in aiming to increase equality and well-being of all individuals in society when our politics is grounded on proper ontology.

So, to hold a naturalised view of impairment does not imply oppression of disabled people. Quite the opposite: ontology based on facts rather than representations is better also in political terms. A view that acknowledges the material basis of impairments is useful and, indeed, necessary for individuals with these conditions because their conditions have a physical grounding that require a physical response. There are cases where people do need the medical model of *impairment;* they need *facts* about the physical consequences of impairment or any other medical conditions they may have (though not all impairments are medical conditions in the sense that they would require medical attention). In plain English, people need tablets, operations, therapies, and other remedies that should be based on medical facts. Millions of competing texts, discourses and representations are not much of a comfort for people who are in pain.

To conclude, there is nothing oppressive in admitting that disability and impairment include both physical and social dimensions. Multiple sclerosis is a medical matter, and the social participation of a person with multiple sclerosis is both a medical and a political matter. In other words, impairment in general is often both a brute fact and an institutional fact, and disability is an institutional fact based on the hierarchy of facts which all ultimately rest on brute facts.

Acknowledgement

We would like to thank Dan Goodley, Katja Kurri and Arto Laitinen for constructive comments on earlier drafts of this chapter.

54 *Simo Vehmas and Pekka Mäkelä*

Notes

1 We understand disability as a social construct in a broad sense including both the material dimensions (i.e., the various socio-economic practices and structures of society that shape people's lives) as well as language, values and ideas that intertwine with the disabling material arrangements.
2 The point presented by Goodley and Rapley is so obvious that it appears to us a bit pointless: we cannot talk about anything at all or express any thoughts without language.
3 Biological laws do not necessarily have to do anything with statistical means. For instance, according to the normal process of development laid eggs develop into an adult fish despite the fact that only in one in a million cases this actually happens. Nevertheless, according to biological laws, this is a normal process.
4 This is, of course, an empirically complicated issue that would deserve a discussion of its own.

Bibliography

Albrecht, G. L. (2002) 'American Pragmatism, Sociology and the Development of Disability Studies', in C. Barnes, M. Oliver and L. Barton (eds), *Disability Studies Today*, Cambridge: Polity Press.

Barnes, C. (1996) 'Disability and the Myth of the Independent Researcher', *Disability and Society*, 11: 107–10.

Barnes, C., Mercer, G. and Shakespeare, T. (1999) *Exploring Disability: A Sociological Introduction*, Cambridge: Polity.

Barnes, C. and Sheldon, A. (2007) '"Emancipatory" Disability Research and Special Educational Needs', in L. Florian (ed.), *The SAGE Handbook of Special Education*, London: Sage.

Baron, S., Riddell, S. and Wilkinson, H. (1998) 'The Best Burgers? The Person with Learning Difficulties as Worker', in T. Shakespeare (ed.) *The Disability Reader: Social Science Perspectives*, London: Continuum.

Barton, L. (1998) 'Sociology, Disability Studies and Education: Some Observations', in T. Shakespeare (ed.), *The Disability Reader: Social Science Perspectives*, London: Continuum.

Best, S. (2007) 'The Social Construction of Pain: An Evaluation', *Disability and Society*, 22: 161–71.

Bogdan, R. and Taylor, S. J. (1994) *The Social Meaning of Mental Retardation: Two Life Stories*, New York: Teachers College Press.

Burr, V. (2003) *Social Constructionism*, 2nd edn, London and New York: Routledge.

Cahoone, L. (2002) 'Introduction', in L. Cahoone (ed.), *From Modernism to Postmodernism: An Anthology*, 2nd edn, Oxford: Blackwell.

Cooper, P. (2001) 'Understanding AD/HD: A Brief Critical Review of Literature', *Children and Society*, 15: 387–95.

Danforth, S. (2000) 'What Can the Field of Developmental Disabilities Learn from Michel Foucault?', *Mental Retardation*, 38: 364–9.

Danforth, S. and Rhodes, W. C. (1997) 'Deconstructing Disability: A Philosophy for Inclusion', *Remedial and Special Education*, 18: 357–66.

Fuss, D. (1989) *Essentially Speaking: Feminism, Nature and Difference*, New York: Routledge.

Goodley, D. (2001) '"Learning Difficulties," The Social Model of Disability and Impairment: Challenging Epistemologies', *Disability and Society*, 16: 207–31.

Goodley, D. and Rapley, M. (2002) 'Changing the Subject: Postmodernity and People with "Learning Difficulties"', in M. Corker and T. Shakespeare (eds), *Disability/Postmodernity: Embodying Disability Theory*, London: Continuum.

Hacking, I. (1986) 'Making Up People', in T. C. Heller, M. Sosna and D. E. Wellbery (eds), *Reconstructing Individualism: Autonomy, Individuality, and the Self in Western Thought*, Stanford, CA: Stanford University Press.

—— (1995) *Rewriting the Soul: Multiple Personality and the Sciences of Memory*, Princeton, NJ: Princeton University Press.

—— (1999) *The Social Construction of What?*, Cambridge, MA: Harvard University Press.

—— (2006) ' Kinds of People: Moving Targets', *The Tenth British Academy Lecture*, 11 April at the British Academy, London: The British Academy. Online. Available HTTP: < http://www.britac.ac.uk/pubs/src/_pdf/hacking.pdf > (accessed 26 March 2007).

Hughes, B. (1999) 'The Constitution of Impairment: Modernity and the Aesthetic of Oppression', *Disability and Society*, 14: 155–72.

—— (2002) 'Disability and the Body', in C. Barnes, M. Oliver and L. Barton (eds), *Disability Studies Today*, Cambridge: Polity Press.

Hughes, P. and Paterson, K. (1997) 'The Social Model of Disability and the Disappearing Body: Towards a Sociology of Impairment', *Disability and Society*, 12: 325–40.

Levine, J. E. (1997) 'Re-Visioning Attention Deficit Hyperactivity Disorder (ADHD)', *Clinical Social Work Journal*, 25: 197–209.

Linton, S. (1998) *Claiming Disability: Knowledge and Identity*, New York: New York University Press.

Mercer, G. (2002) 'Emancipatory Disability Research' in C. Barnes, M. Oliver and L. Barton (eds), *Disability Studies Today*, Cambridge: Polity Press.

Morris, J. (1991) *Pride Against Prejudice*, London: Women's Press.

Oliver, M. (1992) 'Changing the Social Relations of Research Production?', *Disability, Handicap and Society*, 7: 101–14.

—— (2004) 'The Social Model in Action: If I Had a Hammer', in C. Barnes and G. Mercer (eds), *Implementing the Social Model of Disability: Theory and Research*, Leeds: The Disability Press.

Paterson, K. and Hughes, B. (1999) 'Disability Studies and Phenomenology: The Carnal Politics of Everyday Life', *Disability and Society*, 14: 597–610.

Roets, G., Goodley, D. and Van Hove, G. (2007) 'Narrative in a Nutshell: Sharing Hopes, Fears, and Dreams with Self-Advocates', *Intellectual and Developmental Disabilities*, 45: 323–34.

Searle, J. R. (1995) *The Construction of Social Reality*, London: Penguin.

Shakespeare, T. (2006) *Disability Rights and Wrongs*, London and New York: Routledge.

Shakespeare, T. and Watson, N. (2001) 'The Social Model of Disability: An Outdated Ideology?', *Research in Social Science and Disability*, 2: 9–28.

Shildrick, M. and Price, J. (1996) 'Breaking the Boundaries of the Broken Body', *Body and Society*, 2: 93–113.

Stone, E. and Priestley, M. (1996) 'Parasites, Pawns and Partners: Disability Research and the Role of Non-Disabled Researchers', *British Journal of Sociology*, 47: 699–716.

Taylor, S. (1996) 'Disability Studies and Mental Retardation', *Disability Studies Quarterly*, 16: 4–13.

Thomas, C. (1999) *Female Forms: Experiencing and Understanding Disability*, Buckingham: Open University Press.

—— (2002) 'Disability Theory: Key Ideas, Issues and Thinkers', in C. Barnes, M. Oliver and L. Barton (eds), *Disability Studies Today*, Cambridge: Polity.

—— (2004a) 'How is Disability Understood? An Examination of Sociological Approaches', *Disability and Society*, 19: 569–83.

—— (2004b) 'Rescuing a Social Relational Understanding of Disability', *Scandinavian Journal of Disability Research*, 6: 22–36.

Tremain, S. (2002) 'On the Subject of Impairment', in M. Corker and T. Shakespeare (eds), *Disability/Postmodernity: Embodying Disability Theory*, London: Continuum.

Vehmas S. (2003) 'Live and Let Die? Disability in Bioethics', *New Review of Bioethics*, 1: 145–57.

—— (2008) 'Philosophy and Science: The Axes of Evil in Disability Studies?', *Journal of Medical Ethics*, 34: 21–3.

Wendell, S. (1996) *The Rejected Body: Feminist Philosophical Reflections on Disability*, London and New York: Routledge.

Williams, S. J. (1999) 'Is Anybody There? Critical Realism, Chronic Illness and the Disability Debate', *Sociology of Health and Illness*, 21: 797–819.

4 Disability and the thinking body

Jackie Leach Scully

Over the past few decades, political and social changes coupled with medical advances have opened up new spaces for thinking about physical and mental deviations from the norm. Disability today can be framed as an emancipatory movement and minority-rights issue; a biomedical phenomenon; an emergent political identity; a set of social relationships and practices; and as this collection shows, as a topic of philosophical and ethical inquiry. The reconceptualisation of disability within disability studies has made it possible to study impairment as one form of variation among humans, thus joining the general late-twentieth-century trend of attending to *difference* as a 'significant and central axis of subjectivity and social life' (Corker 1999: 630). Taking disability into consideration does not simply introduce a new analytic focus on a form of marginalised identity, however. As well as expanding our knowledge of impairment and its consequences, disability offers new perspectives on issues such as autonomy, competence, embodiment, wholeness, human perfectibility, finitude and limits, the relationship between the individual and the community, all of them notions that 'pervade every aspect' of our lives (Linton 1998: 118), issues with which moral philosophy and bioethics constantly grapple. It recentres the body within philosophical thought.

Ethics and the body

The criticism that the Western philosophical tradition has chronically failed to take embodiment seriously is now well rehearsed. An enduring preference for envisaging the self as a disembodied, decontextualised, ahistorical locus of consciousness means that philosophers talking about moral agents are concerned with agential capacities for rational thought, or with behavioural or (sometimes) emotional characteristics, not with physical features of embodiment. Post-Enlightenment ethical thinking has also tended to interpret the desire for a universalisable ethics as meaning that people are most fairly treated as if they were already indistinguishable in their morally relevant features, as if stripped of the traits that make them different, including their bodily traits. Mainstream moral philosophy thus tends to treat bodies as barriers to rather than sources of moral insight.

In reality, however, moral philosophy and ethics are always concerned with bodies because morality is about behaviour, and behaviour involves bodies. Our basic sense of moral concern reflects an awareness that individuals are vulnerable to each other through their embodied selves, and subsequent ethical theories and rules are abstractions that attempt to regulate what happens when embodied humans interact. Once we start to think of ethics and ontology in this way, an obvious question is whether it is not just the *general* fact of embodiment, but also the *specifics* of body and place, that are significant to individual moral understanding as well.

This makes impaired or disabled embodiment worth closer philosophical attention for more than one reason. For one thing, it has some profound implications for thinking about the nature of human being and identity: If disability is a form of being, rather than a medical condition, what sort of being is it? How exactly does it develop? What relationship does disability have to other social or ontological categories, such as gender, ethnicity or class? Is disability a genuine ontological category, or is it just a useful organising category for a motley collection of odd bodies? And if it *is* an identity, can it ever be anything other than a spoilt one (Goffman 1971) that we are morally obliged to restore to normality if we can, or prevent happening if we can't?

What we really think about bodies that differ from the norm is also ethically important, because our beliefs about normal embodiment become normative. They identify ideal bodies and determine the degree of effort we think it appropriate to expend in order to normalise anomalous ones. In moral philosophy, and specifically bioethics, normative ideas about bodies and body anomalies have particular potency when they inform the frameworks in which quality of life decision are made. 'Quality-of-life' evaluations have enormous moral weight when they form the basis for life-or-death decisions, especially when such decisions have to be made by third parties on behalf of another (end-of-life decisions and prenatal screening and termination for impairment are examples). Yet despite this, the bioethical discussions of such decisions are generally not supported by a clear philosophical theory of the quality of life. In addition, they are based on a number of assumptions including: (1) that we have an adequate grasp of the features of the life being evaluated; and (2) that there is broad agreement about which features are relevant to life quality and how they can be measured. Neither assumption is tenable in the context of impairment and disability: (1) because of the lack of knowledge on the part of those making the evaluations about the realities of life with impairment; and (2) because the subjective experience of impairment or disability may change some of the criteria for gauging quality of life, or their weighting or prioritisation by the individuals concerned (Albrecht and Devliger 1999; Amundsen 2005). In effect, we could say that the experience of impairment or disability modifies the moral understandings of disabled people.[1]

To understand how embodiment affects a person's world requires more empirical approaches than normally taken by moral philosophy. But while empirical work may illuminate the features of life as a particular body, it makes no attempt to say what it is like to *be* that embodiment. This demands a more phenomenological approach. Phenomenology recognises that a subject's sense of self, perceptions and understandings are dependent on how the subject experiences his or her presence in the world; from a phenomenological point of view, presence in the world is an accumulation of everyday bodily events and encounters. If the embodiment is a socially or biologically anomalous one, that fact will affect the nature of the everyday events and encounters, at times very profoundly.

In addressing the strong version of the social model of disability, which views disability as a product of materially excluding social barriers, a phenomenological approach has major flaws. Social models of disability redirect the analytic gaze away from the pathologised individual and towards social practices. The strong social model attempts to sever the link between embodiment and disability by arguing that disability is not about the individual impaired body, but about a stigmatised group being oppressed within a disabling society. Phenomenological philosophy's strategy of paying close attention to the lived experience of being (in) a different kind of body runs counter to this. Hence, social model critics argue that a phenomenological approach places the 'problem' of disability back with the pathologised individual and distracts from the real issue, which is that societies are arranged so as to disable people who are different.

Despite this, scholars within disability studies have argued that a more phenomenological intelligence about disability, understanding the experience of disability from the inside, is an essential part of making ethical and ontological judgements about impairment. Such subjective understanding of disabled experience goes some way towards correcting the long-standing philosophical neglect of the body as an important source of insight into real moral lives. It is not a claim that experiential accounts are the *only* true source material for thinking about disability, nor that a deeper knowledge of disabled experience will rapidly generate a consensus on the meaning and ethics of disability. The disabled body understood through everyday subjective experience can form only a part of the contemporary understanding of abnormality and disability. Other insights, such as the disabled body as typically presented by medical discourse, its representations in popular culture, the understandings of carers and so on, are also necessary contributions to a fuller picture.

The thinking body

Is it possible that having or being a particular kind of body can result in a person acquiring particular moral understandings? Is it further possible that having or being an *anomalous* body can lead to the production of *anomalous* moral understandings? This aspect of the phenomenology of embodiment has not yet received much consideration. Yet it is apparent that at least in *some* circumstances, disabled people have rather different takes on ethical questions relevant to disability than do nondisabled people. Recent and well-known examples would include the arguments against the withdrawal of life support in the case of Theresa Schiavo (Wolfson 2005) or the cases where deaf people express a preference for having a hearing impaired child (Anstey 2002; Johnston 2005; Levy 2002; Parker 2007; Schmidt 2007; Scully 2008).[2] Feminist standpoint epistemology suggests that different social positions provide distinct epistemic perspectives (Harding 1993, 2004; Hartsock 1983), sometimes even an epistemic advantage in perceiving injustices within a situation. What interests me here is the extent to which the experience of anomalous embodiment, as a parallel to the experience of gendered embodiment within feminist theory, contributes to this.

If it is possible that being physically unusual affects a person's moral understandings, it is important for philosophers to identify the processes through which that might occur and the resulting differences it might make. I want now to examine the philosopher Maurice Merleau-Ponty's work, which directly addresses the most primordial interactions between the body and its physical surroundings. Merleau-Ponty's phenomenological approach to the thinking body provides some analytic traction on the impact of bodily variation on moral understanding. In part because of the limited neurological knowledge available in his time, however, Merleau-Ponty ultimately does not provide a satisfying theory of the epistemic consequences of bodily variation, and at this point I turn to recent work in neuroscience that to some degree supports Merleau-Ponty's philosophical claims. Research into what is called 'embodied cognition' provides some substantiation for the idea that both the organic reality of the body and its processes are important to abstract thinking, and hence that different embodiments may have subtle effects on higher order cognition, including thinking about ethics.

Although Merleau-Ponty is usually classed as a phenomenologist, his methodological approach differs radically from his phenomenological predecessors and contemporaries. Brentano, Husserl and Heidegger struggled to get at the truth of being-in-the-world through the knowledge of phenomena but were less concerned with concretising the body as the medium through which phenomena become known. As a result, they downplayed the way that the necessary involvement of the body means that *being-in-the-world* is something more like *being-in-the-body-in-the-world* By contrast, Merleau-Ponty argues that the processes of perception and motility are embodied, and are central to the phenomenological grasp of being-in-the-world (Merleau-Ponty 2002).

Traditional cognitive science and philosophy favour the kind of epistemology in which our knowledge of reality is achieved through the construction of interior mental representations of the world. This epistemology involves the separation of immaterial mind and material body, and a further split between the interior representations of the mind and the world outside. Much twentieth-century psychology, philosophy of mind and cognitive science has relied on a model of the body in the world receiving sensory stimuli, leaving the mind to interpret it and do its best to control the body's acts. The body itself is treated as not of major interest, except at its most extreme as a kind of machine for generating and housing representations of external phenomena.

So, Merleau-Ponty's suggestion that the human body is the *basis* of the mind is a departure from tradition. By saying that the mind is embodied, Merleau-Ponty means that mental life is a function of the kinetic and sensory relations between the body and its setting. Thinking of all kinds emerges as a product of these relations. This product is initially pre-linguistic and precognitive, the 'primary consciousness' seen in our ability to negotiate the world without actively thinking about it all the time. What Merleau-Ponty means by 'mind' is largely this early pre-reflective knowing. Nevertheless, he also holds that the body is the basis for higher-order, conscious rational thought and representation, which is developmentally secondary to embodied preconscious processes. Thought, then, is not a set of propositions structured by a mind distinct from the body: rather, bodily actions or habits make thinking possible in the first place. And so the body and its habitual actions constitute forms of knowledge in themselves about how to be particular kinds of human beings in particular social settings.

Getting a grip on things

Merleau-Ponty's special contribution to phenomenological theorising of the impaired body is a description of the interdependence of the *primary* experiences of embodied human life, that of sensation, perception and motion, which point to how these experiences might then go on to ground thought. Perception is more than the body passively receiving information about the world; it is also how the body inhabits it. Furthermore, there is collaboration between perceptual and motor processes which is best seen, Merleau-Ponty suggests, as one way in which the body has an intentional (that is, object-directed) grip on its physical and social environment:

> my body is geared onto the world [some translations have 'has a grip on the world'] when my perception presents me with a spectacle as varied and as clearly articulated as possible, and when my motor intentions, as they unfold, receive the responses they expect from the world. This maximum sharpness of perception and action points clearly to a perceptual *ground*, a basis of my life, a general setting in which my body can coexist with the world.
>
> (Merleau-Ponty 2002: 292)

For embodied entities, being-in-the-world means constantly striving to achieve the best possible grip on it. Merleau-Ponty locates this process exactly and concretely in the mechanics of sensory input and motor responses. The perceptual milieu instructs bodily orientation, movements and skills. Through engagement in the range of everyday activities, we learn that there are bodily attitudes that give us a 'best grip' on things. For example, most of us learn the stance that keeps us upright and balanced within the gravitational field, just as we also discover by trial and error that there are comportments that help us listen or observe or concentrate. Perception and action are therefore essential collaborators with each other from our first embodied moments. Understanding perception and movement as constitutive of each other in this way, not two distinct functions, dissolves the traditional conceptual split between the mental and the material.

Prelinguistic, non-conceptual content

This phenomenology attempts to expose the world of perceptions and understandings that exist before words or interpretations become possible, or even necessary.

Merleau-Ponty's achievement was to struggle to articulate forms of experience that are by definition hard if not impossible to bring to speech: what is going on for the body, prior to any form of language. Although most philosophy deals in rational thought processes, rational discourse is often inappropriate for the pre-predicative life of consciousness, the primordial layer of experiences that are normally never put into propositional subject/predicate form.

This is important because Merleau-Ponty insists that developmentally early bodily experience is foundational for all kinds of thought. The body is the foundation for the mind because it is the primary spatial and temporal interactions of bodies with their surroundings (perception, movement and actions) that eventually produce more complex cognitive structures that support conscious and symbolic thought, while the level of wordless awareness persists as the organising principle of most of the body's everyday being-in-the-world. Hence in suggesting that cognitive capacities are the developmental spin-offs of accumulated bodily spatiotemporal actions in the material world, Merleau-Ponty concludes that the body is the foundation of imaginative and analytical processes as well. The embodied, non-conceptual content of experience underlies all our subsequent categories, priorities and judgements.

Corporeal schema

Merleau-Ponty used the corporeal or body schema to describe the pre-reflexive sense of the boundaries of the subject's body and what it and its constituent parts are doing. This proprioceptive sense enables us to move and position ourselves without having to think about it. Both psychoanalysis and developmental neurology theorise that the sense of boundedness and bodily self-control that grows throughout early life is linked to the parallel emergence of an integrated psychic sense of self. Before and for a while after birth it is probable that an infant does not possess much of a self/other boundary in terms of its sensations, structures, orientation to other objects and so on. Coherent somatic and psychic identity is painstakingly acquired through the repetition of bodily actions, as initially fragmented perceptions coalesce into a more or less stable sense of self-controlled separateness from other animate and inanimate objects.[3]

The idea of the corporeal schema, assembled through the organisation of tactile, kinaesthetic and proprioceptive inputs, has re-emerged in contemporary neuro-scientific work on embodiment. The scientific literature differentiates between the *body schema*, as a set of sensorimotor processes that operate below the level of awareness, and the *body image*, a culturally derived and usually conscious system of concepts and beliefs about one's body.[4] The two can be distinguished in terms of their availability to consciousness. Body image consists of beliefs and representations, the intentional object of which is the subject's body, whereas the body schema operates below the level of the subject's intentionality (Gallagher and Cole 1995: 371). Because many aspects of body image are conscious and can be put into words, it is amenable to revision – a negative body image can be changed through conscious cognitive work.[5] The body schema, on the other hand, lies outside consciousness (Gallagher 2005). The schema is an interior construction that refers not just to how the body is, but how it is in relation to its surroundings. It therefore supports a dynamic, dialectical epistemology that dissolves the distinction of subject/object. Knowledge of the world and its object components is mediated through the corporeal expressions of action and competences, and these are in turn modified through repeated patterns of encounter with the world.

Embodied mind in neuroscience

Although Merleau-Ponty makes a persuasive *phenomenological* case for the embodiment of mind, he does not take up the question of what sort of mechanism might possibly transform primary sensorimotor experience into higher order thinking. This is true even though he draws extensively on existing psychological, psychoanalytic and, most significantly, neuro-physiological studies to support his philosophical arguments about cognition. Much of his empirical data come from neuropathology, where the effects of disruptions to the standard apparatus inform his philosophical modelling of phenomenological norms. In his later work[6] he is concerned to acknowledge that conceptual forms of knowing are dependent on and have their origins in perception, and he turns his attention to describing the production of higher order functions, such as communication with other people, through and beyond perception (Merleau-Ponty 1964; Sallis 1981), but does not propose a process through which embodiment might determine significant aspects of complex cognition. So while the elaboration of an embodied basis for primary consciousness might be plausible, it is harder to see how to connect this to symbolic thinking, conceptualisation, imagination, memory and so on.

This makes it difficult to make informed suggestions about what kind of difference an *anomalous body* might make to thinking. We could predict that not having standard issue arms and legs, for instance, will result in an unusual orientation of body to its surroundings, establishing and reinforcing slightly variant pathways of sensory input and motor response, and in Merleau-Ponty's phenomenology this would matter for the subject's grip on the world – indeed, whether it is possible to establish an adequate grip at all. But to suggest that this might influence the processes of abstract thought takes things a significant step further.

Over the last couple of decades, support for a so-called *embodied cognition* has been gaining ground within neuroscience. Embodied cognition claims that complex mental processes are founded on the physical interactions that people have with their environments;[7] and this is contrasted with the classic or first generation view which sees cognition as essentially computational and rule-based. A diversity of views on embodied cognition exists, and a comprehensive review of their implications for theorising ethics in disability is beyond what I can do here.[8] Behind all of these views is the idea, familiar from Merleau-Ponty's phenomenology, that both a subject's sensorimotor capacities and the environment combine to facilitate the development of specific cognitive capacities. Early subjective experience of the body interacting with the material world generates neural substrates, which are then available to form the basis for thought and later language. Humans and other primates are born[9] with the basics of a distributed neural network. This is developmentally refined as babies learn about their bodies and the environment, or through 'systematic interactions between tactile, proprioceptive and vestibular inputs, as well as between such inputs and the visual perception of the structure and movements of one's own and other people's bodies' (Berlucchi and Aglioti 1997: 560).

Hence cognition is formed through the influence of constraints that are both intrinsic and environmental. This is a radical break from the view of cognition and consciousness that prevailed in mid- to late-twentieth-century cognitive science, in which a subject's mental events operate pretty much independently of the organic matter, other than neural tissue, of which the subject is composed.

Embodied language

In the embodied cognition thesis, data from a range of cognitive science sub-disciplines are used to support the general hypothesis that aspects of bodily experience structure abstract concepts. But even if cognition cantilevers out from more basic neural structures, that still leaves open the question of how exactly bodies give rise to specifically moral thinking. One intriguing suggestion, which I outline here, is the view that abstract concepts (including moral concepts such as 'autonomy' and 'justice') are understood through embodied metaphor.

Cognitive linguists have long puzzled over the human capacity to understand and use abstract concepts such as those deployed in moral discourse. Although linguistics treats language as an abstract propositional system independent of embodiment, new lines of work present a case for the body, or more precisely the body's sensory and motor experience, having something to do with how people understand certain words and phrases, and how these words and phrases emerge in language to carry their meanings. In this view, conceptual abstraction is not primarily mediated through representations and propositions, but through embodied interactions, especially patterns of bodily actions, perceptions, and manipulations of objects (Gibbs 1996; Johnson 1987; Lakoff and Johnson 1980, 1999, 2002). Briefly, the idea is that in the course of interacting habitually with the world and objects in it, *image schemas* are generated. Image schemas are not mental pictures but a combination of visual, auditory, tactile and kinaesthetic components in 'experiential gestalts' (Gibbs *et al.* 2004: 1192) that give coherence to recurring perceptual and motor bodily experiences. An example that appears frequently in the literature is that of an image schema for *balance* (Gibbs 2005; Johnson 1987). Early physical experiences of balance and disequilibrium, ranging from the obvious (losing one's balance and falling over) to the less so (feeling too cold or too hot, too wet or too dry) give us, it is postulated, a grasp of the meaning of being in balance or being unbalanced.

The claim here is that we understand the non-literal meanings of metaphors not because they are linguistic conventions that we have acquired, but because they have *embodied* meaning for us. I want to emphasise that these theorists do not claim that the body is *all there is* in terms of cognition; social organisations and culture provide frames and constraints, and embodied associations are culturally modifiable. Moreover, the embodied metaphor thesis is not universally accepted by cognitive linguists. Critics say that the available evidence simply does not yet allow us to distinguish a model in which sensorimotor experience is foundational to the understanding of abstract concepts, from one in which the association between particular spatial relationships and those concepts is purely conventional and learned (Glucksberg 2001; Murphy 1996). But *if* it turns out to be the case that people use aspects of their phenomenal experience to structure abstract concepts, then the associated experiential elements (such as the connection of verticality to dominance, or of balance to fairness) are irreducible parts of our basic understanding of them.

The place of variant bodies

From the perspective of disability, the truly striking thing about both phenomenological and neuro-scientific theories is the virtually total focus on normative forms of embodiment. Merleau-Ponty said rather little about non-normative body forms. His work has been heavily criticised by feminist phenomenologists for its gender bias; even his writing on sexuality, a topic which clearly has *something* to do with gendered difference, takes as standard the male embodied experience. Iris Marion Young notes that Merleau-Ponty simply fails to provide any account of the forms of corporeality that are specific to women, such as the gendered experiences of pregnancy or having breasts (Young 2005), while according to Elizabeth Grosz, 'Never once in his writings does he make any suggestion that his formulations may have been derived from the valorisation and analysis of the experience of only one kind of subject' (Grosz 1994: 110). These criticisms of the phenomenological neglect of the gendered body apply equally well to the treatment of other types of phenotypic variance. It must be acknowledged that Merleau-Ponty does engage with impaired embodiment, but apart from a brief discussion of visual impairment in the context of extensions to the corporeal schema it is mostly with a view to clarifying the 'normal' state. He uses neuropathological data, such as the case of the brain-damaged Schneider (Merleau-Ponty 2002: 118–59) to explore some of the consequences of anomalies in perception and neural integration, and he refers to the effect of illness, saying that in disease states the body's intentional arc 'goes limp' (Merleau-Ponty 2002: 157). These are references to illness as a disruption or breakdown of the unified lived body (Diprose 1994: 106); it is not about a different kind of body having a different kind of corporeal schema, one that is as normal and functional to that subject as the 'normal' body is to others. The commitment to establishing a universal phenomenological ontology seems to render phenomenologists unwilling to acknowledge any variation in the primary normative experience for fear of undermining the claim that being-in-the-world can be described in terms of a common primordial perception.

But a phenomenology that dichotomises the experience of being-in-the-world into the normal (the one we focus on) and the pathological (variants that are only interesting for what they tell us about normality) obscures the obvious fact that even fully functioning people are enormously variable in their capacity for certain perceptions or actions. Whenever a 'normal' spontaneous body sense is invoked, we need to keep in mind that this sense operates along something like a continuum with multiple axes. Even in 'normal' people, the smoothly intentional arc of perception and motion that Merleau-Ponty takes as universal and foundational to thinking is often, in reality, awkward, incomplete or flawed. Body phenomenology has not given much attention to this kind of variation, or to the extremes that shade towards the abnormal at both ends of the spectrum of competence.

Currently at least, cognitive science is also vulnerable to this criticism. The data I sketched earlier in support of embodied cognition come from experiments and observations using nondisabled people as experimental subjects. I am not aware of any studies carried out within the embodied cognition paradigm that have yet tried specifically to take into account differences in perceptual and motor experiences that follow from having a body that senses or moves in a different way from the norm. This is a significant gap, precisely because the embodied mind paradigm argues that it's the *particularities* of an organism's embodiment that condition the nature of the experiences that serve as its basis for cognition. If sensorimotor experiences shape the conceptual categories that we are able to construct, they also, in the end, shape how the world appears to us, and the paradigm suggests that changing the particularities of the body then has some effect on cognition. There are one or two brief asides in the literature that point to impairment in principle as a possible source of variation. Van Rompay *et al.* (2005: 347), for instance, comment that 'the embodied interactions of a handicapped person differ substantially from the interactions of those fully mobile'. But apart from exceptions such as these, cognitive scientists have done little to acknowledge that the body of the subject in which they are interested does not necessarily adhere to the standard form.

Ironically, more consideration has been given to the effect on the corporeal schema of the body's habitual association with objects such as tools, clothes, vehicles or jewellery. This does have special resonance for disabled people, many of whom live in long-term association with different assistive devices: canes, wheelchairs, prosthetic limbs, hearing aids, or guide dogs. Experimental psychology and clinical neurobiology have both provided compelling evidence that body schemas can morph to continuously reconfigure the individual's state of being in the world and to include objects that are not organically part of the body. And Merleau-Ponty himself maintained that the body is *not* defined by the boundary of the skin, but extends itself by rendering some external objects as within those boundaries. The corporeal schema is in constant flux to incorporate some and separate off other specific external objects:

> If I am in the habit of driving a car, I enter a narrow opening and see that I can't 'get through' without comparing the width of the opening with that of the wings, just as I go through a doorway without checking the width of the doorway against that of my body. The car has ceased to be an object ... The blind man's stick has ceased to be an object for him, and is no longer perceived for itself; its point has become an area of sensitivity, extending

the scope and active radius of touch, and providing a parallel to sight. In the exploration of things, the length of the stick does not enter expressly as a middle term: the blind man is rather aware of it through the position of objects than of the position of objects through it … To get used to … a stick, is to be transplanted into [it], or conversely, to incorporate [it] into the bulk of our own bodies.

(Merleau-Ponty 2002: 165–6)

Recent work with neuro-prosthetic limbs confirms that interaction with external objects prompts some rewiring of neural connectivity. More strikingly, it also suggests that the external object need not even be in physical contact with the body for this to occur. A group working at Duke University has reported that macaque and rhesus monkeys could learn to control unattached robotic arms by means of brain signals alone, using a brain-machine interface.[10] In May 2005 it was reported that these monkeys showed remodelling of the neural circuits that were used to control their own, attached arms. Neuronal connections appeared to have been shifted so that the monkey's brain could incorporate properties of the robotic arm as if it were another arm. The investigators argued that these results extend the accepted view of brain plasticity to include prosthetics of various kinds: 'Everything from cars to clothing that we use in our lives becomes incorporated into our sense of self.'[11]

Quite how far this can be taken, and especially whether it can be extended to such 'objects' as assistive animals or other persons, are the next questions – unanswerable at present because of the lack of data. There are tantalising hints from some accounts, and a fascinating example is given in the anthropologist Gelya Frank's long-term study of Diane DeVries, who was born with vestigial limbs. Frank writes:

Many of the experiences Diane eventually described did not fit neatly within the conventional concept of the 'body'. For example, Diane's interdependence with others … engendered an intimacy and identification that defied normal definitions of the bounded body. Consider Diane's participation in [her sister Debbie's] learning to dance: 'It's true that there is a Diane within this Diane who can dance, which enabled me to teach my younger sister Debbie. But there's another reason I could coach her so well. [I not only saw her body moving.] I felt her movements in a sense, part of her body (the part I lacked on the exterior) was mine too. So, since I knew how her body moved, I could coach her in dancing.'

(Frank 2000: 124)

If it is true that pervasive sensory and motor pathways provide the basic framework for consciousness, and that bodily experiences generate image schemas that underpin a host of related concrete and abstract concepts, it would be predicted that bodily difference might have unanticipated effects on cognitive processes. Other consequences are also possible, of course. It could be that there is no effect, or the magnitude of difference may be too minor to be noticeable. It could be that the high degree of plasticity and/or redundancy that is so often observed in neural and other biological processes ensures that altered sensorimotor inputs are channelled into common conserved pathways so that the end result, in terms of cognition, is indistinguishable from the norm. At the moment, with the present level of neuroscientific understanding and lack of empirical data, we are simply not in a position to make much of a guess of how much, or what kind, of difference it might make.

If we took the 'differently embodied cognition' argument to the extreme, it could suggest that a person who was unable from birth to make voluntary, repeated bodily actions would also end up unable to *think* in any way as other people do. And this is plainly nonsense. Even given that such impairments are very rare, there is not a shred of empirical or anecdotal evidence to back up such a strong conclusion. People who from birth have a severely compromised capacity for self-controlled movement, perhaps as a result of cerebral palsy or hereditary myopathies, are otherwise cognitively intact. More plausible then is the weaker claim that the corporeal schema of, say, a person with congenital limb anomalies or other kinds of skeletal dysplasia, a conjoined twin, or lifelong wheelchair user, will be different in some subtle but possibly significant ways from the corporeal schema of a person with a standard model body. Whether and to what extent this is true for people with less physically extensive impairments, which have less impact on gross morphology or motor ability, is not a question we can answer at the moment. At first glance, I find it intuitively unlikely that minor variations – congenital deafness, for example, or missing or extra digits – could significantly alter a subject's body schema. And yet personal experience suggests that I orient myself constantly with reference to the sources of sound, and more importantly for me, light, in ways that are subtly unlike the ways of hearing people. I'm certainly not conscious of doing it, but it suggests that my perceptual and motor organisation is responding to environmental cues and working together differently than they do for audio-normals, and it may be that this is true for other anomalous embodiments as well.

What about the effects of anomalous body–environment interactions on higher order cognition? Mark Johnson, one of the first philosophers to take the neuro-linguistic work into the context of ethics, argues that the embodied construction of conceptual metaphor has profound ethical implications. In his book on moral imagination, Johnson (1993) suggests that everyday *moral* thinking is organised through metaphors and semantic frames that are rooted in bodily processes. Under moral thinking he includes a range of processes such as the description of moral situations, the analytical thinking that leads to moral evaluations and judgements, and basic moral abstractions (freedom, duties, rights, action). Rights, for instance, are seen as possessions ('I have this right; you owe me that as a right'). Duties are burdens ('his duties weigh him down; can we take some of the load off?') Rights and responsibilities should be in equilibrium ('with rights come responsibilities'). In the embodied metaphor model, image schemata about verticality and balance generate foundational ideas about the moral worth of balance and equilibrium.

This is reflected in everyday moral discourse as we then speak approvingly about a *balance of power*, or a *well-balanced* argument, or person; fairness is about being *even-handed;* political and intellectual *instability* is to be avoided. Similarly, the embodied value given to being vertical and upright, higher rather than lower, is transferred to the moral domain metaphorically through corresponding phrases: thus a good man is an *upright person*, or *high-minded;* or conversely, *falls* from grace. Someone can *stand on her own two feet*, or conversely has to be *carried by everyone else.*

This has some interesting implications. In essence, the embodied mind and conceptual metaphor theses suggest that in everyday moral thinking, any situation will be conceptualised predominantly through shared metaphors, semantic frames, or narrative structures (Johnson 1993). It would imply that our pre-existing embodied judgements of the morally relevant features of the situation are applied to the very acts of perceiving and describing it. The unthinking use of metaphors in our descriptive and analytical work with moral issues will condition the kind of reasoning we can do about them, and the conclusions we can reach. It is important to be aware of this as a possibility because, in order to be properly alert to the distorting effects of bias, we need to recognise the conceptual frameworks inherited from our social and moral tradition, or (if the embodied cognition thesis is correct) our embodied experience. It also helps to grasp that the same situation can be framed differently according to the choices of metaphor, while different sets of metaphors will have different moral obligations arising from them. The idea that social position has an influence on the way a person perceives and describes events is hardly new; the less familiar idea introduced here is that the biophysical, as well as social, nature of a person's bodied presence in the world has some influence on moral perception and interpretation. Through Merleau-Ponty's primary 'silent consciousness' and the newer paradigm of embodied cognition, it becomes possible to imagine how body shapes, movements and practices take on the felt status of normality. These theories of embodied cognition and cognitive linguistics, then, enable us to propose, even tentatively, mechanisms by which the normative force of specific perceptual or motor experiences lines up behind concepts and linguistic constructions. The embodied, preconsciously encoded nature of these dispositions make them virtually unassailable, at least until presented with an external challenge, such as bodily anomaly.

A second implication is that people who, because of their impairments, fail to embody certain valued metaphors – they are not upright, cannot stand on their own two feet, lack get-up-and-go, and so on – will not be afforded the positive connotations that go along with these approved terms. Of course, these associations are not made consciously, and the vocabulary is not (or very rarely) chosen deliberately to set particular meanings to work. But the unconscious layers of meaning contained within certain words or phrases are potent. In everyday discourse, more of our terminology than we realise carries unspoken statements about our own or others' moral status or competence. Kay Toombs understands this when she says, writing about chronic illness, that

[t]he value assigned to upright posture should not be underestimated … Verticality is directly related to autonomy. Just as the infant's sense of autonomy and independence are enhanced by the development of the ability to maintain an upright posture … so there is a corresponding loss of autonomy which accompanies the loss of uprightness.

(Toombs 1993: 65)

It is worth emphasising that my argument is *not* that having/being an unusual embodiment means that people with bodies that are morphologically or functionally unusual inevitably develop completely unique frameworks of understanding, incommensurable with those of 'normal people'. Nor does it mean that everything worth saying about impairment can be boiled down to a side effect of biological body difference. Trying to separate out the effects *of* impairment and the effects of the social and cultural response *to* impairment is often analytically tricky, but more importantly it often does not reflect the truth of the complex interweaving of effects that takes place. Suppose it is really is the case that pre-reflective moral cognition is mediated through sensorimotor pathways laid down by the body interacting with the environment, and that this happens differently when anomalous interactions are involved. It would remain true that differences in the environment and in the cultural and social milieu are as formative of moral cognition as the unusual morphology or movement itself. Thus there can be no essentialist conclusion here that there is a 'disability mind' or 'disability morality', unlike the minds or moralities of 'normal people'.

What it does suggest is that philosophical work on disability is still hampered by lack of answers to some very basic questions about what it is like to live as/ with an anomalous body. The challenge of unusual embodiment is that it poses hard questions of justification to normative standards, especially to the normative ethical evaluations that are performed from a non-disabled perspective (that is, most normative ethics). I would argue that the philosophical engagement with bodily difference will not make much progress until the database of empirical, experiential and scientific knowledge of it is expanded. And this relies on philosophers, social scientists and life scientists taking an interest in disability as a phenomenon worthy of study rather than a problem to be dealt with.

Notes

1 These points are argued more fully in Mackenzie and Scully (2007) and in Scully (2008).
2 Note that I am not arguing that these positions are necessarily right, only that they exemplify situations where differences in moral understanding between disabled and nondisabled have been observed. It also needs pointing out, of course, that not all disabled people were of the same opinion in the Theresa Schiavo case (which involved a legal battle in 2005 to end the care of a woman in a persistent vegetative state) just as not all deaf people either have or agree with acting on a preference to have a deaf child.
3 Note that Merleau-Ponty did not examine the possibility that the coherent sense of self might be a convenient fiction – something that the infant pulls together out of the

chaos of impressions bombarding it in order to function at all, rather than a reflection of how things really are. Later, Lacan and others of the French psychoanalytic school did develop the idea of the self, or ego, as a cover for a truly fragmented psyche. Less attention has been given to the possibility that the sense of somatic unity is equally factitious.

4 Although Merleau-Ponty has been criticised for inconsistency in his use of terminology, Gallagher and Melzoff (1996) argue that in practice he does sustain a consistent distinction between corporeal image and corporeal schema throughout his work.

5 For example, in psychotherapies of patients with body dysmorphia.

6 Merleau-Ponty's final work, *The Visible and the Invisible*, was left incomplete at his death.

7 For much more detail on embodied cognition and cognitive linguistics, see Pecher and Zwaan (2005), Gallagher (2005).

8 See, for example, Wilson (2002), who identifies six distinct claims about embodied cognition: (1) cognition is situated; (2) cognition is time-pressured; (3) cognitive work is offloaded onto the environment; (4) the environment is part of the cognitive system; (5) cognition is connected with action; (6) offline cognition is body-based – that is, sensorimotor functions that originally evolved to serve action and perception have been coopted for use in the thought processes needed to think about situations and events in other times and places, i.e. imagination and memory.

9 There is debate over whether infants are born with no body image or schema (so that both are acquired as a result of postnatal experiences) or whether aspects of either image or schema are 'innate' – genetic, or generated from very early prenatal experiences. This debate is well outside the scope of this book but can be followed in Gallagher (2005), and references therein. That at least something is present from the outset is supported by evidence that babies can imitate facial and bodily movements and expressions from very shortly after birth, and reports of phantom limb sensations in phocomelic children (that is, with congenital absence of limbs); see Thelen (1995), Thelen and Smith (1994), Berlucchi and Aglioti (1997).

10 Reported on the BBC online news service, 13 October 2003, available at < http://news. bbc.co.uk/2/hi/health/3186850.stm >.

11 Reported on Duke University Pratt e-press, Available HTTP: < http://www.pratt.duke. edu/pratt_press/web.php?sid = 230&iid = 29 > (accessed June 2005).

Bibliography

Albrecht, G. L. and Devliger, P. J. (1999) 'The Disability Paradox: High Quality of Life Against All Odds', *Social Science and Medicine*, 48: 977–88.

Amundsen, R. (2005) 'Disability, Ideology, and Quality of Life', in D. Wasserman, J. Bickenbach and R. Wachbroit (eds), *Quality of Life and Human Difference: Genetic Testing, Health Care, and Disability*, Cambridge: Cambridge University Press.

Anstey, K. W. (2002) 'Are Attempts to Have Impaired Children Justifiable?', *Journal of Medical Ethics*, 28: 286–8.

Berlucchi, G. and Aglioti, S. (1997) 'The Body in the Brain: Neural Bases of Corporeal Awareness', *Trends in Neurosciences*, 20: 560–4.

Corker, M. (1999) 'Differences, Conflations and Foundations: The Limits to "Accurate" Theoretical Representation of Disabled People's Experience', *Disability and Society*, 14: 627–42.

Diprose, R. (1994) *The Bodies of Women*, London and New York: Routledge.

Frank, G. (2000) *Venus on Wheels: Two Decades of Dialogue on Disability, Biography, and Being Female in America*, Berkeley, CA: University of California Press.

Gallagher, S. (2005) *How the Body Shapes the Mind*, Oxford: Oxford University Press.

Gallagher, S. and Cole, J. (1995) 'Body Image and Body Schema in a Deafferented Subject', *Journal of Mind and Behaviour*, 16: 369–90.

Gallagher, S. and Melzoff, A. (1996) 'The Earliest Sense of Self and Others: Merleau-Ponty and Recent Developmental Studies', *Philosophical Psychology*, 9: 213–36.

Gibbs, R. W. (1996) 'Why Many Concepts are Metaphorical', *Cognition*, 61: 309–19.

Gibbs, R. W. Jr. (2005) 'Embodiment in Metaphorical Imagination', in Diane Pecher and Rolf A. Zwaan (eds), *Grounding Cognition: The Role of Perception and Action in Memory, Language, and Thinking*, Cambridge: Cambridge University Press.

Gibbs, R. W. Jr., Costa Lima, P. L. and Francozo, E. (2004) 'Metaphor Is Grounded in Embodied Experience', *Journal of Pragmatics*, 36: 1189–210.

Glucksberg, S. (2001) *Understanding Figurative Language*, Oxford: Oxford University Press.

Goffman, E. (1971) *Stigma*, Harmondsworth: Penguin.

Grosz, E. (1994) *Volatile Bodies: Toward a Corporeal Feminism*, Bloomington, IN: Indiana University Press, and Sydney: Allen & Unwin.

Harding, S. (1993) 'Rethinking Standpoint Epistemology: What Is "Strong Objectivity"?', in L. Alcoff and E. Potter (eds), *Feminist Epistemologies*, London and New York: Routledge.

—— (2004) *The Feminist Standpoint Theory Reader: Intellectual and Political Controversies*, London and New York: Routledge.

Hartsock, N. (1983) 'The Feminist Standpoint: Developing the Ground for a Specifically Feminist Historical Materialism', in Sandra Harding and Merrill Hintikka (eds), *Discovering Reality: Feminist Perspectives on Epistemology, Metaphysics, Methodology, and Philosophy of Science*, Boston, MA: Reidel.

Johnson, M. (1987) *The Body in the Mind: The Bodily Basis of Meaning, Imagination, and Reason*, Chicago, IL: University of Chicago Press.

—— (1993) *Moral Imagination: Implications of Cognitive Science for Ethics*, Chicago, IL: University of Chicago Press.

Johnston, T. (2005) 'In One's Own Image: Ethics and the Reproduction of Deafness', *Journal of Deaf Studies and Deaf Education*, 10: 426–41.

Lakoff, G. and Johnson, M. (1980) *Metaphors We Live By*, Chicago, IL: University of Chicago Press.

—— (1999) *Philosophy in the Flesh*, New York: Basic Books.

—— (2002) 'Why Cognitive Science Needs Embodied Realism', *Cognitive Linguistics*, 13: 245–63.

Levy, N. (2002) 'Deafness, Culture and Choice', *Journal of Medical Ethics*, 28: 284–5.

Linton, S. (1998) *Claiming Disability: Knowledge and Identity*, New York: New York University Press.

Mackenzie, C. and Scully, J. L. (2007) 'Moral Imagination, Disability and Embodiment', *Journal of Applied Philosophy*, 24: 335–51.

Merleau-Ponty, M. (1964) *The Primacy of Perception: and Other Essays on Phenomenology, Psychology, the Philosophy of Art, History and Politics*, Evanston, IL: Northwestern University Press.

—— (2002) *The Phenomenology of Perception*, London and New York: Routledge.

Murphy, G. L. (1996) 'On Metaphorical Representation', *Cognition*, 60: 173–204.

Parker, M. (2007) 'The Best Possible Child', *Journal of Medical Ethics*, 33: 279–83.

Pecher, D. and. Zwaan, R. A. (eds) (2005) *Grounding Cognition: The Role of Perception and Action in Memory, Language, and Thinking*, Cambridge: Cambridge University Press.

Sallis, J. (1981) *Merleau-Ponty: Perception, Structure, Language*, Atlantic Highlands, NJ: Humanities Press.

Schmidt, E. B. (2007) 'The Parental Obligation to Expand a Child's Range of Open Futures When Making Genetic Trait Selections for Their Child', *Bioethics* 21: 191–7.

Scully, J. L. (2006) 'Disabled Embodiment and an Ethic of Care', in C. Rehmann-Sutter, M. Düwell and D. Mieth (eds), *Bioethics in Cultural Contexts*, Dordrecht: Springer.

—— (2008) *Disability Bioethics*, Lanham, MD: Rowman and Littlefield.

Thelen, E. (1995) 'Motor Development: A New Synthesis', *American Psychologist*, 50: 79–95.

Toombs, K. (1993) *The Meaning of Illness: A Phenomenological Account of the Different Perspectives of Physician and Patient*, Dordrecht: Kluwer.

van Rompay, T., Hekkert, P., Saakes, D. and Russo, B. (2005) 'Grounding Abstract Object Characteristics in Embodied Interactions', *Acta Psychologica (Amsterdam)*, 119: 315–51.

Wilson, M. (2002) 'Six Views of Embodied Cognition', *Psychonomic Bulletin and Review*, 9: 625–36.

Wolfson, J. (2005) 'Erring on the Side of Theresa Schiavo: Reflections of the Special Guardian Ad Litem', *Hastings Center Report*, 35: 16–19.

Young, I. M. (2005) *On Female Body Experience: 'Throwing Like a Girl' and Other Essays*, Oxford: Oxford University Press.

Part II
Political philosophy

Part II
Political philosophy

5 Personhood and the social inclusion of people with disabilities

A recognition-theoretical approach

Heikki Ikäheimo

Introduction

What is it to be a person? What is it to be a disabled person? Can impairments compromise someone's personhood, or are we persons completely independently of our abilities? If an impaired individual is not taken seriously as a person by others, does this make one less of a person? Or, is being a person independent of the perceptions and attitudes of others? What role does the oft-stated mission of social inclusion play in considering the question of personhood? This is the cluster of philosophical questions addressed in this chapter.

I begin by clarifying some ways one thinks and talks about what it means to be a person. In particular, I draw attention to one of these views, a view which is rarely clearly articulated yet one which grasps an irreducible and central component of what being a person involves, something I term *interpersonal personhood*. I continue with the contention that to be a person in this interpersonal sense is to be on the receiving end of particular kinds of 'recognitive attitudes' from the part of relevant, concrete others. These recognitive attitudes, as discussed in the third part of this chapter, are responses to psychological features that characterise persons, and they are simultaneously way of attributing 'person-making significances' to their objects. It is these significances that make someone a person in the interpersonal sense, within concrete contexts of social life. In other words, cognitive attitudes form 'I–you relationships', or a 'moral we' between recognisers and recognisees.

I then discuss how particular kinds of impairments can lead to the exclusion of people from *personhood* in the interpersonal sense, even if their 'person-making psychological capacities' are in perfect order. I continue by trying make sense of the much-discussed but relatively unclear notions of 'social exclusion and inclusion', and will argue that one of the important and distinct aspects of social exclusion is precisely that of lack of recognition and therefore exclusion from interpersonal personhood in the concrete contexts of social life. In order to successfully confront this form of social exclusion, we need to understand its nature. This requires that we understand what is involved in leading the life of a person, as a person, among other persons.

Personhood: what is it, and why should we care about it?

What is so special about being a person that we should be interested in it? Simply stated, what distinguishes persons from non-persons? In everyday language, the word 'person' is used more or less identically with 'human' in its meaning. Yet it is easy to think of everyday situations where this is not so obvious, or in other words, situations where the notion of 'personhood' has contours that are independent of the notion of 'human being'. Consider the following case examples of a simple exercise of counting the number of 'persons' present:

Case 1: You are in a room with an average, more or less healthy friend of yours. Count how many persons there are in the room. Quite obviously two?

Case 2: You are in a room with a healthy newborn human child. Count. One or two persons in the room?

Case 3: You are in a room with a human being lacking all higher brain functions due to innate malformations. One or two persons?

Case 4: You are in a room with a friend who has suffered massive brain injury in an accident, and is in an irrecoverable coma. One or two?

Whereas in cases such as 1, there is no problem with counting the number of persons, and no obvious reason to think that there is any difference between counting the persons and counting the humans, in cases such as 2–4, things become quite different. There may be no doubt about the number of *humans* in the room, but there is likely to be uncertainty about the number of *persons* there. It is these and similar problematic cases, which show clearly that our everyday operative and mostly unreflected notion of a person or personhood is not simply the same as our notion of a human being.[1]

What could one then say about whether the humans whose personhood is in doubt (as in Cases 2–4) are in fact persons or not? What is at stake in this question and how do we decide? Or in other words, what is our concept of personhood? Obviously, there are enormous differences between these three cases, but on a general level they have at least one similarity which may explain why there may be a genuine question whether the humans in question are persons: each of the human beings in question lacks central capacities that more average people have. To the extent that this leads you not to consider them as persons, or at least hesitate over whether they are persons, then your implicit or explicit concept of personhood would seem to be what we could call a *psychological concept of personhood*. According to psychological concepts of personhood, advocated by a long line of philosophers, being a person is having psychological capacities that only persons have and that therefore distinguish persons from non-persons.

If you then hesitate over whether to count particular human beings as persons or not, at least one possible reason is that you are not sure whether they have such 'person-making' capacities or not. But a more fundamental kind of hesitation may be at stake as well: even if you were sure that given human beings did not have any of the psychological capacities that you think are distinctive of persons, you might feel very uneasy about concluding that they are not persons. (At least many people that I know would.) If this is so, then it seems that your implicit notion of personhood is not exhausted by merely psychological conceptualisations. The chances are that it includes, in addition to psychological elements, some kind of moral element or dimension. This, I believe, is best grasped by thinking about personhood in terms of *status*.

According to what could be called *status concepts of personhood*, being a person is having some fundamental kind or kinds of moral status that non-persons do not have. Hesitation follows when one believes that a human being is not a person in the psychological sense, but one feels uneasy about judging it/her/him as not a person in terms of moral status. Indeed, it seems that our everyday, usually unreflective and inexplicit, concept of personhood is a mixture of the psychological and the status-concept of personhood, and that this is at least part of what easily makes the question about something's/someone's personhood quite confusing when thinking about problematical cases.

What is it then to have 'person-making statuses', or what exactly are the status-concepts of personhood about? As common as talk of the 'status of a person' is, the notion itself has not received much attention in the philosophical literature. The way I see it, we need to distinguish between at least two different ideas when thinking and talking about person-making statuses, both of which are morally highly relevant. In other words, we need to distinguish between two more precise status-concepts or personhood, both of which may well be in play when someone tries to make up her/his mind about a questionable case of personhood. On the one hand, there is what we can call the *institutional status concept of personhood.* According to this concept, being a person is having some institutionally enforced or enforceable 'deontic' status or statuses.[2] The most commonly mentioned example of this in the literature is the 'right to life'.[3] On the other hand, there is what we can call the *interpersonal status concept of personhood.* This concept is usually not clearly articulated in the literature,[4] but once articulated, it is identifiable as a perfectly familiar everyday phenomenon. Being a person in this interpersonal sense is, roughly speaking, being seen as a person by others. More specifically, it is being seen by others in the light of 'person-making significances' that, in practical or moral terms, distinguish persons from non-persons within the subjective viewpoints of other persons. This 'personifying' way of seeing, or attitude towards, others is what gives them the interpersonal status of a person, and thereby makes them persons in the interpersonal sense in concrete contexts of interaction.

Being seen as a person by relevant others, and therefore having the standing or status of a person in one's encounters and interactions, is obviously of great importance to an individual. So too is, in different ways, *seeing others as persons.* Whether you see something/someone in the light of person-making significances or not makes a massive difference to your way of relating to it/her/him in general. We can begin to grasp this difference, following Wilfrid Sellars, by saying that perceiving and accepting someone as a person is thinking of oneself and the other in terms of a moral community or a 'we'.[5] Or, to use Martin Buber's terms, it is a matter of seeing oneself and the other in terms of an 'I–thou relationship' in contrast to an 'I–it relationship' (Buber 1971). This way of thinking, or its possibility, is in different ways at stake in each of the cases previously mentioned, and in more problematic cases at least an important part of what makes them so complicated.

Returning to the example of Case 2: the point is that you cannot quite establish an I–thou relation with a newborn, at least not yet. But there is usually much anticipation of such a relationship going on in expectant relationships with newborns, and such anticipation by relevant others seems indeed to be a necessary condition of children ever developing into persons who can be full partners in I–thou relationships. Thus, even if it would be inappropriate to see infants in terms of full person-making significance, seeing them practically as non-persons is clearly not an adequate way of relating to them either.

Things are very different in Case 3, where there seems to be no way of establishing an I–thou relationship and thus of thinking of one's relationship to the human being in question in terms of a moral community, not even in the anticipatory sense. Thus, even if the human being in question has a special relation to persons through being someone's child, it is difficult or impossible to see it itself as a person in the interpersonal sense.

Finally, in Case 4, establishing or maintaining an I–thou relationship seems to be simply too late. It may be the memory of and longing for a relationship that once was there, and the sorrow for what has been lost, that make it difficult to admit the fact. We often resort, probably mostly unconsciously, to projections of person-making significances to a body that is to us, as it were, a memorial of a (psychological) person who is no longer with us. Still, on reflection, we understand perfectly well that this projection of person-making significance is only a pale copy of a genuinely interpersonal relationship, where seeing others in terms of person-making significances is not mere projection but rather a *response* to what/whom the other is.

Interpersonal personhood, recognition and the constitution of 'we'

Even if seeing humans in terms of 'person-making' significances is arguably one of the most central elements of our lives with each other, it is not at all obvious what exactly these ways of seeing are. With regard to this, I offer three suggestions, stemming from one way of understanding the recently much discussed Hegelian notion of 'recognition' (*Anerkennung* in German) (see, e.g., Honneth 1995; Ikäheimo 2002; Laitinen 2002; Thompson 2006; van den Brink and Owen 2007). Elsewhere I have argued that in the specifically interpersonal sense, recognition should be understood in terms of attitudes of *taking something/-one as a person* (see Ikäheimo 2002, 2007; Ikäheimo and Laitinen 2007a). This general 'personifying' attitude of recognition has three more specific forms, which, following the analysis by Axel Honneth (1995) with some modification, we can call *respect, love* and *contributive valuing*. Respect, love and contributive valuing are thus personifying attitudes that attribute to their objects person-making significances and thereby make them persons in the interpersonal sense. Let me explain this further.

By '*respect*', we can obviously mean many different phenomena. But here it is a name for an attitude that makes someone a person within the perspective of those who respect her/him. In this more specific sense, respect, as an attitude of taking something/someone as a person is, I suggest, to see something/someone as having *authority* over oneself.[6] Respecting another as having authority over oneself is clearly one of the fundamental attitudes that establish a genuinely interpersonal relationship in which the other has the significance of a person, rather than that of a mere thing. When such an authorisation through respect is mutual, we can talk of *co-authority* of the terms or norms of the relationship. This, it seems, is an essential element of the moral communities or '*we's* that persons form together, and it is part of what makes them persons in the first place.

'*Love*' too can of course mean many things. But as a name for a recognitive attitude it has, I suggest, a very special meaning. Aristotle grasped this long ago by saying that *philia* or love in the central sense of the word is wanting what one takes to be good for someone for his or her own sake.[7] Or in other words, caring about someone's happiness or good life intrinsically. As with respect, love in this simple sense also seems to be one of the fundamental attitudes that establish a genuine I–thou relationship, a 'we' or a moral community between persons, and even more so if love is mutual. Clearly, one of the dimensions of having the standing of a person in the shared life-world of persons, and taking part in genuinely interpersonal relationships, is being someone whose happiness or well-being is taken as intrinsically important by others.

There is a third form of the general recognitive attitude that attributes its receiving object a significance which distinguishes its bearer as a person from non-persons in the viewpoint of its subject. This we can call *contributive valuing*. Contributive valuing of a person is not to be confused with intrinsic valuing in the sense of intrinsic concern for someone's happiness or well-being, i.e. with love. Nor should it be confused with *instrumental valuing*. The emotion of *gratitude* is an illustrative litmus test which helps one to distinguish contributive valuing from instrumental valuing. Arguably, you feel gratitude towards someone if you believe that she/he contributes positively to something you value *and if* you value her/him contributively (or as a contributor). You do not feel gratitude towards someone whom you believe contributes positively to something you value, but whom you value only instrumentally (or as an instrument). To think of an extreme example: to the extent that slave-owners value their slaves instrumentally and not contributively, they feel, or feel that they owe, no genuine gratitude to them. That is, they see them in terms of the significance of an instrument, not that of a contributing person. It seems that part of what it is to be a person in the full-fledged sense of the word is to be valued contributively by others and thereby to be seen as a contributing member of a 'we' of persons worthy of gratitude. (There is more to say about what is required of the contributor for gratitude towards her/him to be an appropriate response, and I will return to this later in the chapter.)[8]

Recognitive attitudes as appropriate responses to claims of psychological personhood

An important aspect of what unites the three recognitive attitudes (respect, love and contributive valuing) and thereby the corresponding person-making significances (co-authority, someone whose happiness has intrinsic value, a contributor worthy of gratitude) is, I suggest, that the attitudes are *appropriate or adequate responses to claims* that beings that are persons according to the psychological concept, or psychological persons, present to each other.[9] This tells us a great deal about the psychological constitution of such beings.

Thinking about respect and co-authority, one only needs to spend a day with a healthy infant to realise how much part of becoming a person involves children presenting others with *claims for co-authority* and to realise how important it is that others respond to them with respect. Children are not machines that follow pre-programmed procedures, nor are they animals that can be simply conditioned to act as others want. Rather, they are beings that, by being what they are and acting as they do, practically *demand* taking an active part in the constant production, reproduction, revision and sanctioning of the norms or terms of the interactions and engagement with others. This is part of the psychological make-up that makes persons persons, and already the earliest interaction of infants is saturated with what I earlier termed *anticipation* of full-blown interpersonal relationships with more or less equal authority or co-authority. As in childhood, so too in adulthood, a *lack of adequate response*, or a *disrespectful response* with regard to claims for respect and authority, is in many ways a serious problem: for the claimant, for the addressee, or for both. The code-slogan of the urban-ghetto 'respect me or die' is one extreme reminder of the constitutive need that people who are psychologically persons have for respect from others and thereby for interpersonal personhood.

With regard to love, its importance likewise informs us about something essential concerning the psychological make-up of persons. In short, it is part of their person-making psychological capacities or features that persons are concerned about their happiness or well-being. In contrast, those animals that are not persons (the 'sentient non-persons') are primarily concerned about the immediate satisfaction of needs. The practical viewpoint of persons is in this sense wider or more inclusive than that of sentient non-persons, and this makes persons also *vulnerable* in a special way. In contrast to the *sentient* vulnerability of sentient non-persons consisting of the possibility of pain or frustration of desire, persons are capable of what we can call *eudaimonistic* vulnerability.[10] A being is eudaimonistically vulnerable to the extent that it is capable of 'happiness and misery', to use John Locke's memorable phrase.[11] A being is so capable to the extent that it values something and can represent to itself both beforehand and afterwards the possibility of the flourishing or failure of what it values.[12] It is the capacity of (psychological) persons to succeed or fail in life, to be or become happy or heartbroken depending on whether what they value flourishes or fails, that presents a particular claim for others. The fully adequate or appropriate response to this claim is to take the happiness of the other as intrinsically important, i.e. to love the person in question. Needless to say, a lack of appropriate or adequate response to this claim by relevant others makes the life of a person in the best case lonely, and in the worst case extremely dangerous.[13]

Finally, it seems to be a very important part of what persons are like psychologically that they have, by default as it were, deeply inbuilt hopes of having something to contribute to the good of others and the hope that others would value them as contributors. This could be seen as a sign of some kind of inbuilt egoism or self-aggrandisement in persons, but there are other ways to understand its inevitability in personal life. As with the needs or claims to be taken as an authority among others and as someone whose happiness is intrinsically important (i.e. for respect and love), the need for or claim to being valued as a contributor also tells of the constitutive dependence of persons on each other. Perhaps contrary to appearance, a claim for contributive valuing is *incompatible* with the claimants being an egoist. We can see this by considering what is required of someone to be an appropriate object of gratitude, which, as I have suggested, is a litmus-test for contributive valuing. Namely, it would be clearly inappropriate to feel genuine gratitude towards someone whose deeds promote something that one values, but who *either* acts unfreely, *or* – and this is decisive – acts freely but without the slightest intrinsic concern for one's well-being or happiness.

The point here is that at least some amount of love towards the beneficiaries has to be among the motives of the contributor for her/him to deserve (or call for) their gratitude. And if gratitude presupposes that its object does not act purely selfishly, then contributive valuing as a precondition or constituent of gratitude does as well.[14] To the extent that it is appropriate to respond with gratitude to a (psychological) person, it is part of that person's psychological constitution to have love for others and therefore to want to contribute, for the sake of those others, toward what they value. This clearly is part of what makes a subject psychologically a person according to our everyday or common-sense notion of personhood.

Altogether, the psychological constitution of persons has a close connection to what (psychological) persons expect to be interpersonally, in each other's eyes. To put this somewhat technically, person-making psychological capacities or features pose to others certain claims, the *appropriate response* to which are recognitive attitudes which attribute respective interpersonal person-making significances and thereby constitute the recognisee's being a person in the interpersonal sense. It is by responding in the appropriate way to each other's claims of psychological personhood that persons form moral communities or 'we's in which they relate to each other in a genuinely interpersonal ways, as Is and thous.[15] This much seems to be universally true of persons, regardless of cultural differences.[16]

Personhood and disabilities

Let us now examine a further example of 'counting persons':

Case 5: You suffer from a physical condition which gives you severe forced movements, makes it difficult for you to communicate with other people in any spoken language, and makes you dependent on a wheelchair to move around and an assistant in daily life. But your mind is as bright as anyone's. Often among more or less healthy persons you have a vivid feeling that you do not fully count as a person.

This, or something like this, is surely a predicament experienced by many people. Yet it remains mostly a silent suffering, one which it is often difficult to bring up and which few people talk about. Since there is hardly a more important task for social philosophy than to give voice to silent suffering, let us continue pursuing this case example.

It is as if you were not included, in the implicit countings or accountings of others in concrete contexts of interaction, among the persons present. It is the way they look at you, the fact that that they talk *about* you rather than *to* you (though they may talk to your assistant). When you try to speak to them, you seldom see the light of understanding illuminating their faces, but more often a humiliating mixture of pity and confusion. Indeed, how would they count, if someone asked them to count the number of persons in a room where you are?

But you are a person, aren't you? Your central psychological capacities are perfectly functional, you are capable of responsibility and authority. You deeply value some things and devalue others, and to the extent that you are only given the opportunity, you do want to contribute something positive to the lives of others. That is, you are clearly a person in the psychological sense. Also, you certainly have the same fundamental rights as any other persons in your society, and are therefore without doubt a person also in the institutional status sense.

Yet regardless of all this, you may have a vivid feeling that you do not fully count as a person. Is it irrational for you to think so? Are you simply mistaken? Or is it perhaps that this way of thinking involves some merely metaphorical, perhaps rhetorically powerful but not philosophically serious, sense of what personhood involves? I do not think so. I believe that the experience of exclusion from full personhood in question is perfectly rational, perfectly literal, and to be taken very seriously. What is actually lacking here is one of the components of what it is to be a person in a full-fledged sense: interpersonal personhood. In other words, what is lacking is that relevant others should see you (at least to an adequate degree) in light of person-making significances, and that you should thereby count in the concrete contexts of interaction with them as a person who has authority, a seriously taken claim to happiness, and/or something gratitude-worthy to contribute. That is, you are not included in the moral communities or 'we's of persons as a person. If anything deserves the name 'social exclusion', then this surely does?

Social inclusion as a solution to social exclusion: what are we talking about?

The terms 'social exclusion' and 'inclusion' are today widely used in disability discourses, social-policy declarations, and elsewhere. Yet, the meanings in which these terms are used are usually not particularly clear. As, for instance, Amartya

Sen notes, in the loosest possible sense, basically lacking anything can be called being 'excluded' from it. Hence one can rephrase, say, lacking adequate nutrition, as 'being excluded from adequate nutrition'. But here the term 'exclusion' adds arguably no new information to what we already know: that someone does not have enough to eat (Sen 2000: part 4). If 'social exclusion' means simply lacking anything one has reason not to be without, then it hardly names a new or useful concept at all.

There are of course more distinct senses of the term as well. The ones that seem to me to grasp something important that is not obviously grasped by many other terms are ones that refer to being somehow a partaker in society, social life or interaction with other persons. Let us say that in this general sense 'social exclusion' means being somehow excluded from *social life*, and 'social inclusion' being somehow included in it. But this is of course still quite vague. Let me suggest a way of being more explicit as to what may be at stake when one talks of inclusion in, or exclusion from, social life. My aim is not to discuss all of the possible interpretations, but only some of them and to concentrate predominantly on what I have been focusing on all along: on interpersonal personhood and the way in which being a person in this sense is being included in social life with others.

I suggest that we can usefully analyse social inclusion in terms of a scheme according to which social inclusion is always a case of some *A including B in C in manner D with the status E*. I will not try to be exhaustive of the values that these variables can take, nor of all their possible combinations, but only spell out some of the combinations which I believe are important to grasp and distinguish from each other. For the sake of simplicity, I will assume that A and B are always individuals or collectives of individuals.[17]

To begin with, note first that the qualifier 'social' in 'social inclusion' seems ambivalent in that it can be understood as referring, at least, to *that in which* B is included (C), to *the way in which* B is included (D), as well as to *the status with which* B is included (E). First, as stated, I assume that (C) *that in which* social inclusion is inclusion is always *social life*. In other words, independently of what values the other variables take, social inclusion is always *inclusion in social life*.[18]

Second, it is useful to distinguish analytically between three different *manners* or ways of inclusion in social life (D): the technical (D1), the institutional (D2) and the interpersonal or social (D3).[19] By technical inclusion in social life (D1), I mean the provision of all the possible material, technical or 'systemic' facilities (or their side effects) which enable persons to take part in social life. In the case of people with disabilities wheelchair-ramps are the simple and obvious example: they enable people using wheelchairs to go or be taken to where other people are, and thereby to take part or be 'included' in social life with them. By institutional inclusion in social life (D2), I mean being institutionally attributed deontic statuses which give one an institutionally enforced position within the social order – paradigmatically rights. Finally, by interpersonal, or social, inclusion in social life (D3), I mean being included in concrete events and contexts of interaction through the attitudes or attention of concrete others who are also partakers in them.

Third, (E), the status with which one is included, is an immensely important factor. What is most decisive here is whether one is included *as a person* or not. For instance, slaves are an important part of the social life of slave-holding societies. Yet, in having no rights, the institutional or deontic status with which they are *institutionally* included in social life (D2) is not that of a person, but, rather, of property. Similarly, it is possible to be included *interpersonally* or socially in social life (D3) by concrete others, yet without the interpersonal status of a person. This is what it is to live among and be attended by people who have no attitudes of recognition towards oneself as a person.[20]

Let us return now to the example of Case 5. In this situation you are technically included, at least in the sense that it is possible for you to be physically present in the midst of social life, you are *institutionally* included *as a person* by having at least the same basic rights as anyone else, and you are interpersonally included in the sense of being attended to by people around you. Yet, to the extent that you are *not* an object of their recognitive attitudes and thus not included interpersonally *with the interpersonal standing or status of a person*, in a very important sense you are still socially excluded. It may be that nothing is more humiliating to an individual than her/his being attended to by others in light of significances other than those of a person, or in other words, being included in social life by others as a non-person.[21]

How is it then that such a predicament can come about and what could be done about it? Why is it that people around you do not respond to the claims of your psychological personhood in adequate or appropriate ways, by having recognitive attitudes towards you? There seem to be two possible explanations. Either they experience your claims to personhood but do not, for some reason, respond to them appropriately. Or they do not even experience your claims as justifiable, at least not clearly enough.

To the extent that the others in question are psychologically more or less 'normal' people, it is somewhat implausible that they could experience the claims that your being psychologically a person presents them with yet be totally unmoved to recognition.[22] It is more likely is that they have a genuine problem in experiencing your claims. The others in question are simply incapable, or insufficiently capable, of experiencing you as psychologically a person, due to your unconventional appearance, the relative difficulty of communication, and their lack of experience.

What is there then to be done in order to fight this radical form of social exclusion which many people with disabilities are all too familiar with? The first thing to do is to identify the problem and to produce lucid ways to talk about it. In this regard, it is important to see that we are not dealing primarily with lack of institutional inclusion in social life in the sense of lack of rights, and consequently, the primary means of fighting the problem is not by demanding more rights. Technical (or practical and technical) means, on the other hand, can be very useful.[23] Any means that help non-recognised people to communicate with relevant others may be decisive in 'getting their claims through', getting others to realise that they are persons whose existence in the social space demands more appropriate responses. Another measure would be to affect the moral imagination of society at large, or at least that of the relevant concrete others in question. Here the task is to enhance the readiness and sensitivity of people to 'really look', to borrow freely an expression from Iris Murdoch (1970: 91), and to really see people with the depicted kinds of disabilities as having similar kinds of inner life to oneself, i.e. as psychological persons. Only to the extent that one really understands and accepts that the other has hopes and claims similar to one's own for respect, love and being valued, can one be moved to respond to these with recognition and thus to enter into a genuinely interpersonal relationship with her/him.

This may sound naively humanist and wishy-washy to many readers. If others around one are blind enough not to understand that they are dealing with a person who just happens to be externally somewhat different from them, why care about such fools anyway? Well, a general answer is that a decent, not to mention flourishing, life as a person is in numerous ways dependent on recognition by the others among whom one lives. Recognition by others and thus interpersonal personhood (or lack of it) intimately affect the development, exercise and consummation of the features and capacities that make us persons psychologically. It is simply impossible to have authority in the social world in which one lives if others do not respect one as sharing authority or co-authority with them. Also, it is at least very difficult for anyone to act in ways that significantly enhance one's own happiness or well-being if others around do not even grasp that one is a person capable of happiness and misery. And finally, finding meaning and communion in one's life by contributing to the lives of others is difficult or impossible if others have no idea that one could have something valuable to contribute and the wish to do so.

This means, among other things, that reacting to a lack of recognition by others by deliberately isolating oneself from others and receding into the private sphere of one's own mind provides at best very limited consolation: the very features that make it the mind of a person, and thus oneself psychologically a person, make one dependent on the recognition of others. Whether one likes it or not, realising oneself as a person and thereby finding fulfilment in life largely depends on others perceiving and accepting us as persons. Because of this, it is always better to respond to lack of recognition and inclusion with action rather than resignation. Full personhood is, to put it mildly, something worth struggling for.[24]

Concluding comments

There are many reasons why talking about the personhood of disabled people is something that may cause worry and unease, not least among disabled people themselves. One of the worries is that once the notion of being a person is separated from that of being human, the conclusion is that disabled people are not persons, or at least not to the same degree that average people are. This, then, opens doors to practical consequences that may be catastrophic or at least a likely source of great misery to people with disabilities.

Even if this worry needs to be taken very seriously, there are certain potential fallacies related to it that need to be avoided as well. For one thing, as to the psychological notion of personhood, no one's psychological capacities will get any better simply by not talking about them. Second, there is no inevitable or automatic inference from psychological personhood to institutional personhood. It is a matter of political judgment and decision to which beings institutional personhood (paradigmatically in the sense of the right to life and perhaps some other basic rights) is distributed, and it is not obvious that the degree of an individual's psychological personhood is the decisive or single criterion on which such a judgment should be based.

As to what I have called interpersonal personhood, or the interpersonal component of what it is to be a person in a full-fledged sense, it is simply a fact that many disabled people suffer from lack of it. This is not something we should keep silent about, but something we should try to change. Since there is so much talk about 'social exclusion and inclusion' today, it would be politically wise to point out loudly and clearly the radical ways that people will remain socially excluded simply because of lack of adequate recognitive response by relevant other people in their social environments. It is only when this form of exclusion becomes an explicit part of the public imagination that effective remedies can be expected.

To conclude with a difficult question, what, then, are we to make of the interpersonal personhood of people whose person-making psychological capacities are not as developed as those of average people, yet, who do not lack them altogether? Well, within the limits of their capacities, they obviously *should* have the possibility to enjoy life among respecting, loving and valuing others who, by having such attitudes, enable and support them in leading their lives as fully as they can as persons among other persons. That intellectually disabled people live among and are supported by others whose sensitivities for 'really looking' are cultivated in sharing life with them is also the best possible guarantee that they will be considered with full seriousness on the institutional level. And I would contend that this is as much true of people whose psychological capacities are congenitally limited, as of those whose capacities have become so due to illness, accident or old age.

Acknowledgements

My thanks are due to Ming-Chen Lo and the editors of this collection for their helpful comments. Simo Vehmas' paper 'The Who or What of Steve' (Vehmas 2007) was an important inspiration for me in writing this piece.

Notes

1 Sometimes counting persons is used as an example of a completely untheoretical and unspecific everyday way of using the term 'person'. Yet, counting persons already clearly involves commitment to some notion of what distinguishes persons from non-persons, i.e. commitment to some, however vague, concept of personhood.
2 I take the notion of 'deontic status' from Searle (1995). In brief, it means a status that is collectively or institutionally created. Rights and duties, but also legal or moral 'protections', are cases of deontic status. For a more detailed discussion of the relevant notions of status, see Ikäheimo (2007).

3 See, for instance, Tooley (1972) who stipulates that being a person is simply the same thing as having what he calls 'a serious right to life'. See also Feinberg (1980) who, like many others, distinguishes between 'descriptive' and 'normative' notions of personhood. Feinberg's notion of descriptive personhood corresponds to what I mean by 'psychological personhood'. His notion of 'normative personhood' conceives personhood basically as a right-status, and Feinberg presents a useful catalogue of possible ways in which the right to life can be argued to be grounded in person-making psychological capacities. My notion of 'status-personhood' is broader than Feinberg's notion of normative personhood in that the former covers not only rights- (or duty-) statuses (or 'deontic statuses'), but also statuses that persons occupy 'in each other's eyes' as a function of attitudes of recognition that they have towards each other. In other words, unlike Feinberg, I distinguish between *institutional* status-personhood and *interpersonal* status-personhood.

4 See, however, Spaemann (2007). For criticism of Spaemann, see Ladwig (2007).

5 Sellars (1962: Chapter VII). To be exact, Sellars seems to have in mind only *institutional* status-personhood in my sense. I believe, however, that his idea of the moral community or 'we' as essential for taking something/someone as a person is in fact better grasped by the notion of *interpersonal* status-personhood.

6 See Brandom (1999), who emphasises the importance of mutual authorisation through attitudes of recognition for the existence and content of social norms. What Brandom calls 'recognition' is according to my Honneth-inspired model only one of the attitudes of recognition, the one that I call 'respect'.

7 See Vlastos (1980). A somewhat parallel account of the importance of love (mainly of oneself) for personhood is Frankfurt (2004).

8 It is a commonplace that persons need each other and that *therefore* instrumentalising others is an inevitable part of life. This 'therefore' is, however, fallacious since not all valuing of persons for their contributions is instrumental valuing. Much misguided cynicism about the human condition is due to the general confusion of contributive with instrumental valuing.

9 This is what we propose in Ikäheimo and Laitinen (2007a). I say more about this in Ikäheimo (2007), which contains in general a more systematic presentation of the multi-componential way of thinking about personhood utilised in this text. See also Laitinen (2007) for a related, yet somewhat different, way of conceiving the difficult concept of personhood.

10 By making this distinction I do not mean that it is a matter of either/or. All of the person-making psychological capacities or features come in degrees, and therefore the difference between sentient and eudaimonistic vulnerability is also one of degrees. The word 'eudaimonia' comes from Greek and was used by Aristotle as a name for the overarching good, happiness or good life, which all persons strive for.

11 See Locke (1997: Book 2, Chapters 25, 26). There is some circularity in the formulation that persons are concerned about their happiness, and that this is what makes them capable of happiness. I have no space to address this issue here, but I do not think the circularity in question is vicious.

12 Compare Frankfurt (1988: 83): 'A person who cares about something is, as it were, invested in it. He *identifies* himself with what he cares about in the sense that he makes himself vulnerable to losses and susceptible to benefits depending upon whether what he cares about is diminished or enhanced.'

13 Just consider the precariousness of life among people to whom one's happiness is a matter of complete indifference or to whom it has merely instrumental value, as a dispensable means for profit-making. Much security can be achieved by institutionalised rights and duties, as the liberal tradition of political philosophy teaches, but very little respect for these would be guaranteed if the parties were purely self-interested and had no intrinsic concern for the well-being of others. For instance, Mead (1962: Chapter 37) and Parsons (1990: 330) agree on this.

14 This is so if a particular model of the emotions is true, as I take it to be. According to this model, an emotion with content p consists of (1) some kind of appraisal or 'pro-attitude' towards content p, and (2) the belief that p is, or is not, the case. Conceived in

terms of this model, we can then usefully understand A's emotion of gratitude towards B as gratitude that B contributes freely and out of (some) love for something that A values. That B contributes freely and out of (some) love for something that A values is thus here the content p, and contributive valuing is the pro-attitude towards p that together with the belief that p constitutes the emotion in question. Note that this does not yet say what exactly distinguishes contributive valuing from instrumental valuing. The same p can of course be an object of instrumental valuing too. Yet, instrumental valuing of p together with the belief that p does not constitute gratitude.

15 The expression 'claims of personhood' is ambiguous of course. What I mean by a 'claim *of psychological* personhood' is a claim *to interpersonal* personhood. Thus recognition in the sense of taking someone as a person, and thereby attributing to her the interpersonal status of a person, is the appropriate response to such a claim. There are other 'claims of personhood' as well, most prominently the claims *to institutional* personhood (i.e. to being given the institutional status of a person), and the claims *of institutional* personhood (i.e. to being treated by others according to one's institutional status as a person).

16 In other words, the above discussed intertwinement of psychological capacities and appropriate responses seems constitutive of *a general form of life* – namely that of persons – within the perimeters of which we judge different cultures as different specifications of this general form.

17 More loosely, the logical subject of social inclusion (A) can also be understood as something other than real individual subjects or collectives of such subjects. In this looser sense one can talk of, say, institutions or social arrangements including or excluding some people. I will not discuss this further here, but will assume that social inclusion and exclusion are, on reflection, always analysable as something 'between people'.

18 This is, for instance, the general sense in which Nancy Fraser and Axel Honneth talk about 'social inclusion' in Honneth and Fraser (2003). Compare also the UPIAS definition of disability: 'Disability is the disadvantage or restriction caused by a contemporary social organisation which takes no or little account of people who have impairments and thus *excludes* them from the *mainstream of social activities* [emphasis HI]' (in 'Fundamental Principles of Disability' by The Union of the Physically Impaired Against Segregation and The Disability Alliance, reprinted in Oliver 1996: 22).

19 That this is an 'analytic' distinction means, roughly, that these three ways are in real life usually closely connected.

20 I deliberately identify 'social' with 'interpersonal' to mark the difference to 'institutional'. One of the central ideas behind this way of looking at things is that interpersonal attitudes of recognition are the foundation of sociality or 'social life'.

21 'Objectification' and 'reification' are also words often used for this phenomenon. As to the latter, see Pitkin (1987) and Honneth (2008).

22 One way of describing 'psychopaths' is to say that while they are capable of experiencing others as psychological persons, they are, however, incapable of being moved by the claims that the others being psychological persons present them with, and thus unable to take others as persons in the interpersonal sense. In other words, psychopathy is incapacity for recognition.

23 See Bach (2002) for an insightful criticism of attempts to understand social inclusion exclusively in terms of rights. Bach also emphasises lack of recognition as a form of social exclusion, which cannot be remedied simply by more inclusion in the sense of more rights. Talk of technical means for inclusion and talk of rights are not completely separate things, since the availability of adequate technical means (say, ramps, means for helping communication, etc.) may be institutionalised as subjective rights.

24 Obviously, collective political organisation is of prime importance. The risk that political organisation needs to avoid, however, is that it remains for its participants predominantly a source of consoling peer-group-recognition, accompanied with shared but self-deceptive denial of the recognition by 'the others' having any significance.

Bibliography

Bach, M. (2002) *Social Inclusion as Solidarity: Rethinking the Child Rights Agenda*, The Laidlaw Foundation. Available HTTP: < http://www.laidlawfdn.org/cms/file/children/ bach.pdf > (accessed 28 August 2007).

Brandom, R. (1999) 'Some Pragmatist Themes in Hegel's Idealism: Negotiation and Administration in Hegel's Account of the Structure and Content of Conceptual Norms', *European Journal of Philosophy*, 7: 164–89.

Buber, M. (1971) *I and Thou*, New York: Free Press.

Feinberg, J. (1980) 'Abortion', in T. Regan (ed.), *Matters of Life and Death*, New York: Random House.

Frankfurt, H. (1988) 'The Importance of What We Care About', in H. Frankfurt, *The Importance of What We Care About: Philosophical Essays*, Cambridge: Cambridge University Press.

—— (2004) *Reasons of Love*, Princeton, NJ: Princeton University Press.

Honneth, A. (1995) *The Struggle for Recognition: The Moral and Political Grammar of Social Conflicts*, Cambridge: Polity Press.

—— (2008), *Recognition: A New Look at an Old Ideal*, Oxford: Oxford University Press.

Honneth, A. and Fraser, N. (2003) *Redistribution or Recognition? A Political-Philosophical Exchange*, London: Verso.

Ikäheimo, H. (2002) 'On the Genus and Species of Recognition', *Inquiry*, 45: 447–62.

—— (2007) 'Recognising Persons', in H. Ikäheimo and A. Laitinen (eds), *Dimensions of Personhood*, Exeter: Academic Imprint.

Ikäheimo, H. and Laitinen, A. (2007a) 'Analysing Recognition: Identification, Acknowledgement and Recognitive Attitudes Between Persons', in B. van den Brink and D. Owen (eds), *Recognition and Power: Axel Honneth and the Tradition of Critical Social Theory*, Cambridge: Cambridge University Press.

—— (eds) (2007b) *Dimensions of Personhood*, Exeter: Academic Imprint.

Ladwig, B. (2007) 'Das Recht auf Leben – nicht nur für Personen', *Deutsche Zeitschrift für Philosophie*, 55: 17–39.

Laitinen, A. (2002) 'Interpersonal Recognition: A Response to Value or a Precondition of Personhood?', *Inquiry*, 45: 463–78.

—— (2007) 'Sorting Out Aspects of Personhood', in H. Ikäheimo and A. Laitinen (eds), *Dimensions of Personhood*, Exeter: Academic Imprint.

Locke, J. (1997) *An Essay Concerning Human Understanding*, New York: Penguin Books.

Mead, G. H. (1962) *Mind, Self and Society*, Chicago, IL: University of Chicago Press.

Murdoch, I. (1970) *The Sovereignty of Good*, London: Routledge & Kegan Paul.

Oliver, M. (1996) *Understanding Disability: From Theory to Practice*, Basingstoke: Macmillan.

Parsons, T. (1990) 'Prolegomena to a Theory of Social Institutions', *American Sociological Review*, 55: 319–33.

Pitkin, H. (1987) 'Rethinking Reification', *Theory and Society*, 16: 263–93.

Searle, J. (1995) *The Construction of Social Reality*, London: Penguin.

Sellars, W. (1963) 'Philosophy and the Scientific Image of Man', in R. Colodny (ed.), *Frontiers of Science and Philosophy*, Pittsburgh, PA: University of Pittsburgh Press.

Sen, A. (2000) *Social Exclusion: Concept, Application and Scrutiny*, Social Development Papers No. 1. Asian Development Bank. Available HTTP: < http://http://www.adb.org/ Documents/Books/Social_Exclusion > (accessed 28 August 2007).

Spaemann, R. (2007) *Persons: The Difference Between 'Someone' and 'Something'*, New York: Oxford University Press.

Thompson, S. (2006) *Political Theory of Recognition: A Critical Introduction*, Cambridge: Polity Press.

Tooley, M. (1972) 'Abortion and Infanticide', *Philosophy and Public Affairs*, 2: 37–65.

van den Brink, B. and Owen, D. (eds) (2007) *Recognition and Power: Axel Honneth and the Tradition of Critical Social Theory*, Cambridge: Cambridge University Press.

Vehmas, S. (2008) 'The Who or What of Steve', in M. Häyry, T. Takala, P. Herissone-Kelly and G. Arnason (eds), *Arguments and Analysis in Bioethics*, New York: Rodopi.

Vlastos, G. (1981) 'The Individual as an Object of Love in Plato', in G. Vlastos, *Platonic Studies*, Princeton, NJ: Princeton University Press.

6 Disability and freedom

Richard Hull

Introduction

This chapter presents disability as an issue of human freedom. It discusses the relation between ability and freedom. Many traditional approaches to freedom tend to rule out the idea that disability can be seen as an issue of human freedom. However, it is suggested here that such approaches render freedom quite meaningless in a lot of contexts when, in real life, the importance of freedom stems from the fact that we consider it to have practical meaning. A model of freedom is introduced that links freedom quite closely with ability, capturing the idea that freedom has practical meaning. Using that model, disability can be seen as an issue of freedom. Indeed, it is shown that the kinds of things denied to people who are disabled are important basic freedoms that are conditional to the enjoyment of many other aspects of life. An advantage of such an approach is that it gives disabled people's claims for better social provision more moral force. That is, they are claims for the provision of important basic freedoms, which any notion of a just and fair society ought to take seriously. Such an approach, then, renders our concept of freedom more inclusive, meaningful and applicable, enabling theorists to more adequately articulate the remediable hardships endured by many members of our community.

The relation between ability and freedom is discussed below. I will claim that inability and thus that disability is a source of unfreedom. Rawls' worth of liberty distinction stands in the way of making that claim. I will argue that, in allowing for almost entirely worthless freedoms, Rawls' concept of freedom is very minimalist and quite meaningless to a lot of people. Instead, we should concede that social and natural contingencies are among the constraints *definitive* of liberty rather than merely being constraints definitive of its worth. It follows from this that disabled people's claims for rights are very well grounded. They are claims for the provision of important basic freedoms.

To make a start, something should be said about the concept of disability that will be assumed in the rest of the chapter. It is an idea of disability that is intended to bridge the often perceived divide between the medical and social models of disability. I have argued elsewhere that disability generally involves the concerns of both the medical and social models (Hull 1998: 199–210; 2007: 19–28) – that impairment can and does cause disability but, more often than not, disability has a lot to do with particular social structures and arrangements. And while it is useful (especially in the context of thinking about social justice) to distinguish disabilities that result primarily from impairment from those that result primarily from a socially inadequate or discriminatory response to impairment, disability often involves a highly complex interplay of impairment and social factors. As Jonathan Glover so ably puts it, 'disability involves a functional limitation, which (either on its own or – more usually – in combination with social disadvantage) impairs the capacity for human flourishing' (Glover 2006: 9).

With the above in mind, the basic argument to be explored here runs as follows. We cannot be said in any meaningful sense to be free to do that which we are unable to do. People with physical impairments are often unable to participate in a range of activities that other people are able to participate in, largely due to social structures and arrangements. Therefore, they cannot be said to be free to so participate. Moreover, given that the restrictions of freedom are usually socially determined and remediable, we should seriously question the justice of a society where such conditions endure.[1]

This argument runs up against (at least) two important contributions to political theory that tend to dominate discussion: the idea of negative liberty and Rawls' theory of justice. Both of these contributions will be criticised in the light of ethical issues concerning disability.

Miller notes that negative liberty theory 'has become the dominant view of liberty in practical politics and in the writing of many liberal theorists' (1991: 8). On the negative view, freedom is seen as natural and given. The absence of interference by external agents is sufficient for its realisation. In addition, negative liberty theorists tend to stipulate what can count as an external obstacle to freedom. For example, natural obstacles are said not to violate freedom; 'I am rendered unfree by an obstacle, only if that obstacle is imposed by another person, not if it is the result of an accident of nature' (Gray 1991: 22). As noted above, it is also held that obstacles have to be external to impede freedom. It can be argued from this sort of position that people with physical impairments face natural and internal obstacles which, by definition, cannot impede their freedom. A physical impairment is said to reduce 'the agent's ability, but not her freedom' (ibid.: 22).[2] I want to suggest that such an approach is unhelpful.

How we view the relation between freedom and ability will be important in determining which approach to freedom we find most sensible. For example, the negative position allows that one can be free to do that which one is unable to do. As we have seen, it limits what can count as a constraint to freedom. Through doing this, many incapacities are denied the moral severity that attaches to claims about freedom. As a result, social injustices can be obscured by the claim that we are all free in a negative sense. That claim is evasive and renders freedom rather mysterious.

To illustrate, let us suppose that I want to jump from a second-floor balcony, perform a somersault and land without any pain or injury. I want to live out some unrealised gymnastic fantasy. Let us assume that there is no law against making such a jump. Let us also assume that I do not own a property with a second-floor balcony. I must thereby pay a levy to a capitalist friend of mine to gain access to her balcony. Assuming that I can pay the levy, whether I can perform my jump, somersault and painless landing will very much depend upon my ability as an acrobat. If I cannot afford to pay the levy, I will be unable to perform my jump whether or not I can perform it painlessly. Now in what sense can I be said to be free to perform my jump, somersault and painless landing if (1) I am physically unable to do it even though I can afford it; (2) I am physically able to do it but cannot afford it; or (3) I am physically unable to do it *and* cannot afford it? Moreover, in what sense can my liberty be said to be equal to that of a rich acrobat? I could be said to be conceptually or legally free to jump from the balcony without suffering pain or injury on landing but, in reality, this freedom means very little to me unless I am also *able* to make such a jump – physically and financially. We should ask, then, why a freedom that means almost nothing[3] to me is called a freedom, given the political and moral connotations of the word.[4]

We might argue instead, for example, that if those with particular needs can do less with their wealth because of the cost of their need, then to say that their liberty remains unaffected is insensitive. However, John Rawls challenges that sort of claim. He asserts that 'The inability to take advantage of one's rights and opportunities as a result of poverty and ignorance, and a lack of means generally, is sometimes counted among the constraints definitive of liberty. I shall not, however, say this, but rather I shall think of these things as affecting the worth of liberty' (Rawls 1972: 204).

Applying this to the above example, I may lack the physical and/or fiscal means to perform my somersault without inducing serious injury upon landing but I am indeed free to complete the jump without pain, it is just that that freedom is worth very little to me. Here, then, meaningless or worthless freedoms are freedoms nonetheless and while this enables Rawls to maintain that we can all be said to be free, it is not at all obvious that we should accept such a minimalistic conception of human freedom. If we should reject such a conception, then we should likewise reject the idea that we can all be said to be free.

Rawls' idea is that his first principle of justice guarantees equal liberty for all and his second principle maximises the worth of liberty to the least advantaged.

> Freedom as equal liberty is the same for all; the question of compensating for a less than equal liberty does not arise. But the worth of liberty is not the same for everyone. Some have greater authority and wealth, and therefore greater means to achieve their aims. The lesser worth of liberty is, however, compensated for, since the capacity of the less fortunate members of society to achieve their aims would be even less were they not to accept the existing inequalities whenever the difference principle is satisfied ... Taking the two principles together, the basic structure is to be arranged to maximise the worth to the least advantaged of the complete scheme of equal liberty shared by all.
>
> (ibid.: 204–5)

This passage does not seem to mention the influence of natural contingencies such as physical ability on freedom, although one would think that they would be considered as partly comprising the possession or 'lack of means generally'. This is hardly surprising given that Rawls doesn't take sufficient account of the impact that natural contingencies can have when considering who is the worst off in society. The passage does, however, deny that wealth directly affects freedom (and natural contingencies clearly affect what we can do with our wealth). Wealth is only said to affect the worth of our freedom.

Pogge construes Rawls' conception of the worth of freedom as a function of three components:

> the public recognition of certain basic freedoms ... their protection ... and the means at one's disposal ... Let us say that the first component determines (formal) legal freedom; that the first two components together determine effective legal freedom (Rawls: freedom); and that all three components together determine worth of freedom or ... worthwhile freedom.
>
> (Pogge 1989: 128)

Pogge argues that, while the third component is dealt with by the second principle of justice, the first principle governs both of the other components, 'reflecting the realisation that basic rights and liberties protect our freedom only insofar as they are themselves well-protected, that is, upheld and enforced' (ibid.: 128).

Asserting that Rawls' lexically prior first principle of justice is attempting to guarantee effective legal freedom means that we are granted more than paper freedoms under that principle. An example of a paper freedom would be where I have the right to do x and you forcibly stop me from doing x. My right to do x is not effective in this case, even though on paper that right is guaranteed. The significance of Rawls' first principle guaranteeing effective legal freedom is that you will be prevented from forcibly stopping me; my right to do x will be protected. However, excluding the third component (the means at one's disposal) from the first principle of justice entails that, while effective legal freedom amounts to more than paper freedom in one sense, it amounts to *no more* than paper freedom in another. That is to say, if I have the right to do x but I cannot afford to do x, my right to do x is still legally effective even though I cannot do x. So, Rawls' first principle ensures that you cannot hold me back but it permits that my situation *can* hold me back. A very possible consequence of this theoretical position, as Pogge aptly notes, is that the integrity of our person would be protected against violence while – at the very same time – it could collapse through deprivation of food and shelter (ibid.: 145). If we are uncomfortable with such a position, we must ask whether Rawls is right to attach so much more importance to effective legal freedom than he does to worthwhile freedom.

Pogge argues that the rationale behind attaching overriding importance to effective legal freedom is that, even though it is the case that the extent to which one is in a position to enjoy one's freedoms is a function of one's wealth and income, without publicly recognised and effectively enforced basic rights, the enjoyment of the correlative freedoms is altogether out of the question (ibid.: 130). We can question, however, whether those in the worst off position in society would always have reason to want an extension of their effective legal freedoms instead of some increase in their means to be able to enjoy them. As Pogge notes, Rawls needs to show both that for each basic liberty, L, having L is lexically more important than having the means for enjoyment of the freedom L protects, and that having L is lexically more important than the means for the enjoyment of *any* first principle freedom (ibid.: 131). This entails that he would have to deny the following possibility:

> that a greater gain in the worthwhile freedom of the poor would result from an improvement in their income and education (enabling them better to take advantage of their existing basic rights and liberties) than from additional legal rights (whose effect on their worthwhile freedom may be rather slight so long as they remain poor and uneducated).
>
> (ibid.: 132)

Yet Rawls does indeed seem to deny such a possibility when he states that 'a departure from the institutions of equal liberty required by the first principle cannot be justified by, or compensated for, by greater social and economic advantages' (1972: 61). Rawls takes the basic liberties of citizens to be, 'roughly speaking':

> political liberty (the right to vote and to be eligible for public office) together with freedom of speech and assembly; liberty of conscience and freedom of thought; freedom of the person along with the right to hold (personal) property; and freedom from arbitrary arrest and seizure as defined by the concept of the rule of law.
>
> (ibid.: 61)

Contra Rawls, it is at the very least insensitive to suggest that those that are lacking social and economic opportunities would or should prefer, say, an extension of their rights of assembly to some help with their heating, clothing or mobility costs. Rawls' insistence on the pre-eminence of the basic civil and political rights and liberties constitutes a denial of the fundamental role that *basic social and economic needs* actually play in a human life (Pogge 1989: 133). We should not accept such a denial.

Rawls' theory runs into these difficulties because lexical priority is assigned to a principle that guarantees more than paper rights in one sense (effective legal freedom) but guarantees no more than paper rights in another (no minimum worth of liberty). Such a position fails to sufficiently acknowledge the impact that social (and natural) contingencies can have on our freedom. Imagine that, by some stretch of the imagination, jumping from a second floor balcony suddenly became a fundamental liberty. Let's say jumping from high places was deemed to have a vital role in self-development, indeed, the higher the better. I think that it is unlikely that we would choose to be assigned a new first principle right to jump from a third floor balcony (that we lack the physical and/or fiscal means to perform) in preference to being given the money to gain access to a second floor balcony and to undergo the training, if required, to *actually jump*. However, Rawls asserts that the idea of incorporating a guaranteed minimum of means at one's disposal into the first principle of justice is superfluous. 'Whatever the merits of this suggestion, it is superfluous in view of the difference principle. For any fraction of the index of primary goods enjoyed by the least advantaged can already be regarded in this manner' (Rawls 1982: 73; Pogge 1989: 136). While this is obviously the case in an ideal situation, where the difference principle is satisfied, it is not in a non-ideal situation,[5] for example, where the first principle of justice is yet to be satisfied. So, a possible strategy for Rawls is to emphasise the design priority (in ideal situations) of the first principle of justice while denying the implementation priority of it (in non-ideal situations) (Pogge 1989: 136).

Although it is a possible strategy for Rawls to restrict the lexical priority of his principles of justice to ideal theory, it is not a strategy that he seems to adopt.

> Viewing the theory of justice as a whole, the ideal part presents a conception of a just society that we are to achieve if we can. Existing institutions are to be judged in the light of this conception ... The lexical ranking of the principles specifies which elements of the ideal are relatively more urgent, and the priority rules this ordering suggests are to be applied to *nonideal* cases as well ... Thus while the principles of justice belong to the theory of an ideal state of affairs, they are generally relevant.
>
> (Rawls 1972: 246; Pogge 1989: 136)

We are still left, then, with the uncomfortable possibility that 'meeting basic social and economic needs will in nonideal contexts take second place to the establishment of basic liberties (which could hardly be enjoyed by those whose basic needs remain unmet)' (Pogge 1989: 139).[6] That we are left with such a possibility suggests that Rawls is wrong to attach so much more importance to effective legal freedom than he does to worthwhile freedom. Indeed, on this alternative view, Rawls is wrong to state that the fundamental liberties are always equal.

We need not accept such a limited idea of human freedom as that expressed by Rawls via his first principle of justice. It is the claim that a worthless freedom is a freedom nonetheless that lands Rawls with the difficulties outlined above. Such a claim fails to sufficiently recognise the impact of social and natural contingencies on human lives. It could be said to be a rather misleading portrayal of 'freedom', for it allows one to hold that everyone in society is equally free while some may not be in a position to meet their basic social and economic needs, a fundamental prerequisite for a minimally worthwhile human life (ibid.: 146). Using the term in this way does not seem to match the moral gravity that is usually attached to it. Yet this is, in effect, what Rawls does. Due to the fact that *worthlessness* is not ruled out, effective legal freedom is a very minimal and potentially meaningless concept of freedom which in turn renders the claim that we should have a right to the most extensive total system of equal basic liberties a rather empty gesture.[7]

The arguments so far suggest that the worth of liberty distinction, as Rawls draws it, is mistaken. Instead, it should be acknowledged that, in order to mean-ingfully describe something as a freedom, some degree of worth must be pres-ent. That is to say, social and natural contingencies should be seen as among the constraints *definitive* of liberty.[8] A freedom would then have to be to some extent worthwhile or realisable so to be articulated as such. Given that at least *some* degree of worth would thereby be stipulated, the worth of liberty distinction would then become operative so to determine the *degree* of worth of a given freedom. If this were to be acknowledged, it would follow that those whose basic social and economic needs remain unmet cannot be said to be free. It would follow, in turn, that the claim that the fundamental liberties are always equal is false.

Hitherto, it has been contended that a concept of liberty would do well to be more sensitive to the influence of both natural and social contingencies on free-dom. This is best done by abandoning the blanket assumption of negative liberty coupled with the worth of liberty clause as Rawls articulates it. Rather, a concep-tion of justice should be sensitive to the influence of natural and social contin-gencies on freedom. This is consistent with Feinberg's point that constraints to freedom can be internal (for example, compulsive desires or ignorance) and also negative (such as poverty or a lack of strength). He argues that, once we realise this, we can dispense with the positive-negative liberty distinction.

> A constraint is something – anything that prevents one from doing something. Therefore, if nothing prevents me from doing x, I am free to do x; conversely, if I am free to do x, then nothing prevents me from doing x. 'Freedom to' and 'freedom from' are in this way logically linked, and there can be no special 'positive freedom' to, which is not also a 'freedom from'.
>
> (Feinberg 1973: 13)

It is appropriate, then, to make a distinction between legal freedom and a more inclusive or realisable freedom and to acknowledge that realisable freedom is con-ditional upon ability, whether physical, fiscal or both.[9] This ensures that worthless freedoms in the Rawlsian sense are clearly demarcated from realisable freedom and lends support to the intuitively appealing idea that we cannot be said in any meaningful sense to be free to do that which we are unable to do.

The example of a person in a wheelchair at the bottom of a flight of stairs will illustrate how freedom is inextricably linked with ability if the concept is to have any meaning to the agent to whom it is meant to apply. Let us assume that the person in a wheelchair is unable to climb stairs. However, on the negative con-ception of liberty she is free to do so. Freedom here means very little to the agent due to their inability to realise it. Contrast this with a person in a wheelchair at the bottom of a ramp. She is, on the negative conception, free to move up the ramp and this freedom is realisable in so far as she *can* move up the ramp. The difference between the two freedoms in this case is immense and remains unaccounted for by the negative model. The former freedom is not only worth very little; it is not a freedom in anything like the same sense as the latter. It is more fitting, then, to make a distinction between legal or hypothetical freedom and realisable freedom. If one is legally free to do x but unable to do x, one is only legally free. If one is legally free to do x and able to do x, freedom is realisable. Likewise, if one is effectively prohibited from doing x but able to do x, one has no freedom and only hypothetical ability; and if one is effectively prohibited from doing x and unable to do x, one has neither freedom nor ability. Thus, a legal or hypothetical freedom cannot be realised without ability and ability cannot be realised without freedom.

While the importance of legal or hypothetical freedom should be acknowledged given that it is a condition of freedom's realisation, it is realisable freedom that is the stuff of value. Worthless freedom is rarely subject to demand. Rather, it is the idea that freedom has practical manifestation that explains why it means such a lot to us – why it is cherished, fought for and taken away as a punishment. In the interests of our concept of freedom matching up with the value we place on our freedom, then, freedom should be recognised as being conditional on ability.[10] To claim that x is free to do y when x is unable to do y can be said to be a manoeuvre lacking substance. It renders freedom relatively meaningless to a lot of people in a lot of contexts. Equating freedom with ability on the other hand is more sympathetic to our intuitions with regard to the value of liberty and encourages that the term is no longer used as a potentially insensitive conceptual veneer.

The idea that freedom cannot be realised without ability has further ramifications in that it admits that there can be many more constraints on an agent's freedom than simply 'external impediments of motion'. Whatever hinders our ability, by implication, hinders our freedom. Exclusion at the point of definition as to what counts as a hindrance is no longer justifiable.[11] In the light of this, we can see that negative liberty theory only articulates part of what it really means to be free. An alternative and more comprehensive definition of freedom is provided by Gerald MacCallum, who argues that underlying both positive and negative conceptions of freedom is the same concept of liberty. He expresses this in the triadic formula; 'x is (is not) free from y to do (not do, become, not become) z' (1991: 102). His formula attempts to elicit as simply as possible what freedom is without prior judgement as to what freedoms are important or what counts as unfreedom. It follows from this that 'differences of opinion over liberty, turn on different interpretations of what (for the purposes of freedom), counts as an agent, a constraint or an objective' (Gray 1991: 12). And the arguments so far suggest that inability should count as a constraint upon freedom. When we are free in the meaningful sense of the word, we are necessarily free to do something whether we do it or not. To do something requires that we are able to do it. Therefore, inability is a source of unfreedom.

Given that inability is a source of unfreedom, disability can be seen to be a source of unfreedom. Disabilities arising from impairments can be seen as restrictions of ability and thus freedom, due to functional limitation. Likewise, disabilities resulting from social arrangements like the widespread failure to provide ramps, for example, can be seen as restrictions upon freedom.[12] Applying Mac-Callum's formula, it seems fairly uncontroversial that a person with an impairment should count as an agent, that economic, political, social, legal, environmental and interpersonal barriers or failures should count as constraints, and that the living of a rough approximation to normal early twenty-first-century life should count as an objective. It is the latter restrictions of freedom that are especially important to political theory given that they are socially determined. The situation is alterable, if not eradicable. By implication, then, our theoretical position should account for the fact that people with impairments have their freedom limited in a variety of ways and that this unfreedom is to a significant extent socially determined. Moreover, it should provide a justification as to why the situation is not altered to increase the freedom of people with impairments.

Before we can begin to question why we do not bother to alter a socially deter-mined situation of limited freedom, that the corresponding freedoms are worth bothering about has to be established. One of the consequences of recognising the dependency of being free to do something on the ability to do it is that the sphere of unfreedom is broadened. Although it can now be asserted, for example, that a person in a wheelchair at the bottom of a flight of stairs is not free in any mean-ingful or practical sense to climb them, it can also be said that neither am I free to wear the Eiffel Tower, jump half a mile into the air or drink fine wine on Jupiter tonight. As a result, the argument might run, the idea of unfreedom is cheapened; it no longer counts for the same as it did under the negative Rawlsian conception. Negative liberty theory rules out superficial claims to unfreedom at the point of definition. I am not unfree to drink fine wine on Jupiter tonight because nobody is stopping me. However, as we have seen, it also rules out many serious incapaci-ties as being concerns of human freedom. In the interests of not doing this, the sphere of unfreedom has been broadened. However, this need not entail that all unfreedoms are as serious as each other and, by implication, that all objectives are of equal value. Rather, it is a question of deciding which freedoms we should be able to enjoy and which abilities we should be free to exercise.[13]

Certain activities are valued over others and the freedoms facilitating their exercise are of corresponding importance. For example, work, travel, social inter-action, education, sport and shopping seem to be valued a lot more than wearing the Eiffel Tower, jumping half a mile into the air and drinking fine wine on Jupiter. This goes some way to explain why offices, roads, bars, schools, football stadi-ums and shopping centres are in greater evidence than lightweight Eiffel Towers, rocket-powered Wellington boots or flights to Jupiter. We have deemed such activities, rightly or wrongly, to be of value and the corresponding freedoms to be worth facilitating and protecting. To be unfree to do these things is thus more seri-ous than to be unfree to do other more superficial or ridiculous things. Moreover, it is clear that the kinds of freedoms denied to people who are disabled are indeed those that are generally deemed by society to be worth granting and protecting. Given this, to argue that people with impairments should continue to have their freedoms limited with regard to education, employment, travel, leisure and social interaction would be either hypocritical or more than a little discriminatory.

Furthermore, the kinds of freedoms denied to people who are disabled are important basic freedoms upon which the enjoyment of other valuable or more superficial freedoms is conditional. Freedoms with regard to housing, education, health, employment and travel, for example, are foundational to the experience of other freedoms as well as being highly valued in themselves. Without them, we could not even entertain the thought of, say, rocket-powered Wellington boots. Nor would there be much left of social and professional life as we presently recognise and enjoy it. Thus, the fact that these freedoms are freedoms upon which so many other pursuits depend entails that to be denied them will have a considerable impact on people's lives. By implication, the continuation of such a state of affairs should be seen as a very serious social and political issue.

Given, then, that the kinds of objectives that disabled people are unfree to pursue are the kinds of objectives that society considers to be worthwhile to be free to pursue, we urgently need to ask why such freedoms are not facilitated or protected in these cases. That such freedoms are conditional to the enjoyment of many other freedoms makes the question all the more important. Political theorists are increasingly recognising the importance of disabled people's legitimate and compelling claims. Denying those claims the moral force that attaches to claims about freedom can only be detrimental to that process.

Acknowledgements

I am very grateful to James Dwyer, John Rogers, Brian Smart, Hillel Steiner and Jonathan Wolff for their comments on earlier drafts of this chapter.

Notes

1 For a much more lengthy version of this argument (with extended application) see Hull (2007: Chapter 3).
2 Gray (1991: 22). However, many problems facing disabled people are indeed external, that is, they are social and environmental and are not secured by functional limitation. Thus, it should be possible to establish disability as an issue of freedom using the traditional negative model.
3 This is not to deny that effective legal freedoms can have some meaning. Suppose I was an old and uneducated black person in the American South. The end of legal segregation in university education might mean a lot to me, even if I were unable to study because, say, I was too old. Here, though, that the end of legal segregation might mean a lot to me would seem to be conditional on the expectation that others will indeed be *able* to study. Thus, while meaning can be derived from effective legal freedoms, freedom tends to mean a lot more if it is realisable, even if not to oneself at a particular point in time. I am very grateful to James Dwyer for this example.
4 Although the liberty at stake here could hardly be said to be fundamental, the example illustrates the kinds of constraints faced by those on the least receiving end of natural and social inequalities.
5 Rawls' assertion would not be true with regard to ideal theory if his conception of justice were to take natural primary goods more fully into account, for his difference principle does not attend to the fact that some need more resources to take the same advantage of their social primary goods as others. While this is an important criticism of his theory of justice, it is not a criticism internal to that theory, since he does not take full account of natural primary goods. If he did, then so arguably would his difference principle. It is worth noting also that the idea being discussed, of incorporating a guar-

anteed minimum of means at one's disposal into the first principle of justice, could be adjusted so as to be more sensitive to natural as well as social inequalities.

6 Pogge (1989: 139). Other strategies open to Rawls are discussed in depth by Pogge. It is sufficient here to note that Pogge shows that either they do not work or that they do not sit comfortably with the rest of his theory.

7 Daniels (1975: 279) makes a similar point when he argues that 'equality of basic liberty seems to be something merely formal, a hollow abstraction lacking real application, if it is not accompanied by equality in the ability to exercise liberty'. Moreover, the fact that Rawls' first principle commands so much attention serves to reinforce the point that we generally take freedom to mean and entail something substantial.

8 See also, with respect to economic factors, Daniels (1975).

9 Van Parijs (1995: 4) similarly argues that 'Both a person's purchasing power and a person's genetic set up, for example, are directly relevant to a person's real freedom ... real freedom is not only a matter of having the right to do what one might want to do, but also a matter of having the means for doing it.'

10 In a similar sense, Sen (1987: 36) writes about 'capability'. 'Capabilities ... are notions of freedom, in the positive sense: what real opportunities you have regarding the life you may lead.'

11 This could be seen to go against Van Parijs' position. He writes that 'the class of desires that could therefore count as freedom-restricting according to the view of real freedom that is here being proposed does not include all desires that would be regarded as freedom-restricting if one of the "positive" conceptions of freedom had been adopted' (1995: 24). An example of what is not included is a desire that diverges from some normative view about what a person ought to desire. However, I do not think that such a desire should be ruled out as freedom-restricting at the point of definition. Rather, the idea that some desires might be freedom-restricting should be open to debate. Indeed, one might argue (while at the same time acknowledging the danger of such an argument) that some tendencies, for example, toward paedophilia or religious extremism, are worth trying to liberate people from.

12 For a more comprehensive discussion of disability resulting from impairment and disability resulting from social arrangements, see Hull (1998: 199–210) or Hull (2007: Chapter 2).

13 This seems to be what Williams (1987: 100–102) envisages when he writes that:

> 'one has to put some constraints on the kinds of capability that are going to count in thinking about the relation between capability on the one hand and well-being or the standard of living on the other ... I think that it is difficult to avoid taking into account the notion of something like a basic capability ... we shall also have to bear in mind that we cannot simply take without correction the locally recognised capacities and incapacities, opportunities and lack of opportunities, because in some cases the question of what is recognised will be ideological ... We have to correct the local expectations of what count as relevant opportunities and lack of opportunities in the light of general social theory and general ethical criticism of these societies.'

Bibliography

Daniels, N. (1975) 'Equal Liberty and Unequal Worth of Liberty', in N. Daniels (ed.), *Reading Rawls*, Oxford: Blackwell.

Feinberg, J. (1973) *Social Philosophy*, Englewood Cliffs, NJ: Prentice Hall.

Glover, J. (2006) *Choosing Children*, Oxford: Oxford University Press.

Gray, T. (1991) *Freedom*, Basingstoke: Macmillan.

Hull, R. (1998) 'Defining Disability: A Philosophical Approach', *Res Publica*, 4: 2.

—— (2007) *Deprivation and Freedom*, London and New York: Routledge.

MacCallum, G. (1991) 'Negative and Positive Freedom', in D. Miller (ed.), *Liberty*, Oxford: Oxford University Press.

Miller, D (ed.) (1991) *Liberty*, Oxford: Oxford University Press.

Pogge, T. W. (1989) *Realising Rawls*, Ithaca, NY: Cornell University Press.

Rawls, J. (1972) *A Theory of Justice*, Oxford: Oxford University Press.

—— (1982) 'The Basic Liberties and Their Priority', in S. McMurrin (ed.), *The Tanner Lectures on Human Value*, Vol. III, Salt Lake City, UT: University of Utah Press.

Sen, A. (1987) *The Standard of Living*, Cambridge: Cambridge University Press.

Van Parijs, P. (1995) *Real Freedom for All*, Oxford: Clarendon Press.

Williams, B. (1987) 'The Standard of Living: Interests and Capabilities', in A. Sen (ed.), *The Standard of Living*, Cambridge: Cambridge University Press.

7   Disability, non-talent and distributive justice

Jerome E. Bickenbach

[T]o criticize inequality and to desire equality is not, as is sometimes suggested, to cherish the romantic illusion that [people] are equal in character and intelligence. It is to hold that, while their natural endowments differ profoundly, it is the mark of a civilized society to aim at eliminating such inequalities as have their source, not in individual differences but in [social and political] organization.

(Tawney 1931: 62)

Introduction

Theories of justice are about what members of social and political communities are entitled to. Justice theories are distinguished in part by the ground or rationale for the provision of entitlements: the need for commensurate and proportionate punishment or praise for *corrective justice;* the need for fair or equal apportionment of resources, welfare or opportunities for *distributive justice;* and the need for fair play, dignity and respect for *procedural* (or *relational*) *justice.* Viewed separately, these entitlements may be allotted in terms of one or several of these rationales; or the allocation that one form of justice requires another may, in the circumstances, prohibit or limit. Tawney's seminal vision was that inequality of income, status and respect (the inequality that truly matters to us) does not flow inexorably from natural differences between people but is a product of the way we organise society: the inequality that is morally deplorable is not 'inequality of personal gifts, but of the social and economic environment' (Tawney 1931: 50). This insight creates an account of justice that merges all three kinds of justice – or rather, one in which corrective and procedural justice are means towards the single goal of egalitarian distributive justice.

Tawney's insight is familiar to disability scholars (though its age belies the ubiquitous labels of 'new paradigms' and 'the new social model'). This includes the underlying perception that the disadvantages of disability are brought about, not simply by the underlying impairment, but as well by social and political institutions. If we broaden Tawney's scope somewhat, and include cultures, attitudes, the built environment, expectations of normality, and so on, we have the essence of the so-called social model of disability, variously described (see e.g., Amundson 1992; Bickenbach 1993; Hahn 1988; Oliver 1986; Saflios-Rothschild

1970; UPIAS 1976; Wright 1983). Here too is the expressed rationale for anti-discrimination law and policy, as embodied in the Americans with Disabilities Act (1980), its predecessors and worldwide successors. Finally, and from the perspective of analysing disability as a demographic variable (like age, sex or ethnicity), for the purposes of describing and measuring the impact of disability on the population, the insight is implicit in current epidemiological models of disability (Altman 2001; Fougeyrollas 1995; Nagi 1965; WHO 1980), including the most recent found in WHO's *International Classification of Functioning, Disability and Health* (WHO 2001) (Bickenbach 1999).

So why revisit Tawney? One reason is that his talk of 'natural endowments' and 'personal gifts' – which we will return to below – appears to support those who, under the rubric of the social model of disability, argue that the disadvantages of disability are entirely or mostly a product of social and political arrangements and have little or nothing to do with underlying impairments. Some disability advocates have expressed doubt that a theory of distributive justice must include entitlements to resources designed to correct or ameliorate the impact of impairments, not because these resources are not required, but because such a justice claim is grounded in the medical model in which disability is primarily viewed as an impairment or functional incapacity.

Anita Silvers in particular argues that this focus on impairments is both demeaning (as it implies that people with health problems are inferior and need to be fixed) and ignores the salient social fact – which the Tawney insight strongly endorses – that the morally deplorable disadvantages that people with impairments face are the result of stigmatisation and discrimination, not from underlying differences in 'natural endowments' (Silvers 1994). On the other side, disability scholars like Tom Shakespeare (2006) object to the social model's refusal to accept that impairments themselves disadvantage people, seemingly moving the centre of gravity of disability scholarship and politics away from Tawney's insight. So, on this debate, Tawney's insight is still current.

The second reason to go back to Tawney is that his blunt statement of the 'inner' and the 'outer' sources of inequalities raises a thorny issue for theories of justice in general, and disability theory in particular. Since it is vital to put this issue clearly, with full regard to both its nuances and its potential pitfalls, I want to begin with a few matters of interpretation so that the insight can be better situated within the disability critique of theories of distributive justice.

Background to Tawney's insight

Although perfectly apt, it remains a somewhat trivial objection to Tawney that the 'inner'/'outer' distinction is simplistic. In an important sense it is: we are ecological entities; the world shapes us just as much as we shape the world. Even at the foundations of our biological being – our genetic make-up – we are buffeted and moulded by evolutionary and environmental forces. And our individual and collective actions return the favour, with ever more dire consequences. If 'inner' and 'outer' suggest a dualism of soul and body, or mental and physical, then as a materialist I am the first to reject the distinction as nonsense. Nonetheless, it remains a useful heuristic. Without denying the fundamental interactive relationship between the 'inner' and the 'outer', we can and should distinguish between ontological levels or planes of experience or whatever, roughly characterised as that which is intrinsic to us as biological and psychological entities and that which forms our habitat, our physical, interpersonal, social, cultural and political environment.

Still, Tawney's expression of the distinction is not helpful. On one side, he uses phrases that are not equivalent: 'character and intelligence', 'natural endowments', 'personal gifts', and 'individual differences'. A cursory reading might suggest he is distinguishing between differences a person can be held responsible for ('character and intelligence') and those that are outside of her control. But that can't be right (although it hints at matters we will return to) since he then speaks of 'natural endowments' and 'personal gifts' which suggests a distinction between attributes one is born with and those one acquires. But surely he does not want to ignore individual differences brought about by life experiences, such as lowered intelligence because of nutritional deprivation, disease, accident, or violence. On the other side, Tawney only speaks of 'social and political organization', which leaves out a vast range of external or extrinsic sources of human differences. Do we include climate, or population density, or other geopolitical factors here or not?

Yet, fundamentally Tawney's insight is easily understood: a social commitment to equality does not demand that all individual differences be equalised, only those disadvantageous differences that are caused by the social and economic environment. We would not be unfaithful to his insight if we elaborated both sources of human difference in a modest way. We can assume that it is 'individual difference' that is the operating notion here, which would generally include all physiological and psychological functional capacities and traits. Thus, by 'character', Tawney might be thought to have in mind such inner human resources as industry, ambition, self-discipline, optimism, emotional stability, creativity, and energy, and by 'intelligence' he surely would be willing to include all talents, skills, and capacities, mental and physical, innate or acquired.

It would be equally fair to Tawney's insight to expand and elaborate the other side of his dichotomy. Though he is only interested in 'social and political organization', all manner of 'external' or 'environmental' factors can influence how one's life is led, or, how one's panoply of intrinsic traits plays out in the world. Some features of the physical environment – time, gravity, and basic physical properties – are outside of the control of social and political institutions. Others are controllable, but at great cost – population distribution, climate control, resource availability and distribution – and others still are increasingly amenable to social and political institutional control – city planning, public health promotion and prevention, discrimination, access to resources. The level, kind and feasibility of social and political control over external or extrinsic sources of differences are huge issues, but nothing is gained conceptually by whittling down the domain of these sources from the outset.

Once we appropriately elaborate the domains of intrinsic and extrinsic sources of human difference, Tawney's insight remains and is strengthened. It becomes the framework for an action plan of social justice: We must remove, modify or otherwise alter all those extrinsic sources of human inequality that are within the control of our social and political institutions. Those extrinsic factors that are realistically out of our control but produce individual differences may require a compensatory state response, in the form of additional social resources to compensate the individual for limits on his or her capacity to participate in basic human and social activities. Whether achieved by direct action (altering the environment) or compensation, equality does not demand that people themselves be 'made the same' or 'equalised' (whatever that would mean). People are different, and that is a good thing generally speaking.

Of course, this is an insight, not a theory. A great deal more needs to be said about what it is that does need to be equalised (access to primary, social goods, resources, welfare, marginal utility, opportunities, capabilities), and something has to be said about how much disparity in advantage is unjust, given that scarcity of social resources and competing demands on them.

Happily, my interest here does not require me to develop Tawney's account of justice, or find a place for him in the tableau of theories and theorists debating theories of distributive justice and the demands of egalitarianism. My interest is to look afresh at Tawney's insight, so elaborated, in light of the disability critique of theories of justice, and raise a concern, not unknown in the justice literature, that disability theorists have not, I believe, properly acknowledged. The concern I have in mind flows from the observation that Tawney's insight applies with equal force to *all and any form* of inequality of advantage, as long as it is amenable to redress by social and political organisation. But first, we need one more refinement of the insight.

It's all about equality

On the face of it, Tawney's insight does not entertain the prospect of 'correcting' or improving all differences in natural endowment or individual capacity, let alone arguing for a social obligation to do so. Human capacities in every domain – intelligence, creativity, concentration, emotional stability, physical strength and coordination – spread out over a continuum. People are different. Tawney may have assumed that – as the phrase 'natural endowments' suggests – this is just 'the hand one is dealt' (although if so, his insight would become rather trivial). Obviously he would be sympathetic to the view that stigma and social exclusion based on perceptions of human difference need to be removed, as these are examples of differences created by the social environment. But what about the intrinsic differences themselves?

If we elaborate Tawney's insight in the manner suggested above, and use impairments as the focus, the question is, would he have argued that justice, and a social commitment to equality, require that – where possible, and to the extent possible – intrinsic inequalities should be corrected or their impact on a person's participation in everyday domestic and social life be ameliorated or compensated?

In other words, how should we characterise a *failure* of social and political institutions to provide resources to correct or ameliorate impairments, to lessen their impact on a person's overall performance in life activities and quality of life? Would this be, in Tawney's eyes, an inequality that has its source, not in individual difference *per se*, but in social and political organisation? Of course it would. Individual differences need not be equalised, but they do create certain needs when they are painful, functionally limiting or get in the way. Unmet need is a socially created inequality, not an individual difference, so long as – we must quickly add – it is possible and feasible to meet these needs by a redistribution of resources. Of course the issue here is not merely unmet needs, but unequally unmet needs. If all unmet needs were ignored, equally, then social inequality may not be created (especially if a compensatory scheme were in place to soften the blow of unmet needs). The morally deplorable sense of inequality is one in which needs are both created, unmet, and thereby worsen unequally, because of social and economic arrangements. There is every reason to think, given the overall argument of his book, *Equality*, that Tawney would wholeheartedly adopt this position.

Yet, to apply Tawney to disability it is crucial to understand his phrase 'such inequalities as have their source … in [social and political] organization' as referring, not merely to discrimination, stigma and other active forms of inequality creation, but also, the absence of structures, or the failure of organisations, to attempt to ameliorate or compensate for the other side of the interaction, namely impairments.

Let us agree, then, that Tawney's invidious inequalities have their source both in active adverse responses from social and political institutions – stigma, prejudice, social exclusion – and passive non-responses, in the form of a failure to respond to the needs created by impairments by providing relevant resources to eliminate or ameliorate the impact of impairments on a person's social participation, or when the needs so created cannot possibly or feasibly be ameliorated, then to provide useful compensation.

As it happens, most societies in the developed world acknowledge and respond to both forms of inequality. Medical, rehabilitative, educative and assistive technology and other forms of accommodation in housing, transportation and communication services are provided to improve or ameliorate limitations in functional capacity. And social assistance, workers' compensation, short- and long-term disability pensions, and an array of other income replacement schemes attempt to compensate individuals whose impairments have affected their capacity to work. These measures, however adequate or rationally administered, are examples of measures motivated by distributive justice.

On the other hand, anti-discrimination laws address the consequences of stigma and stereotyping associated with disability. As anti-discrimination laws and policies are responses to past practices of inequality, they are examples of the application of corrective justice. However, as has been persuasively argued by several scholars of the Americans with Disabilities Act 1980 (in particular, Bagenstos 2000, 2003; Stein 2003), the doctrine of 'reasonable accommodation' adds a redistributive dimension to these laws inasmuch as it requires reasonable accommodations in public, employment and educational settings by way of a response to prior discriminatory practices.

Thus, as Wasserman has remarked (1996, 1998), impairments are relevant to social justice in two different ways: as functional deficits and social markers. Some social responses view impairment as functional deficits that get in the way of a person's social participation; others emphasise the social stigma and other obstacles to full participation that disadvantage people with disabilities. As functional deficits, impairments create needs for services, resources and accommodation, calling up distributive justice; and as forms of social stigma, neglect and misunderstanding that have harmed persons with justice, the response – to try to undo the harm that has been done – calls for corrective or compensatory justice. Wasserman believes, rightly in my view, that since impairments are 'fraught with social meaning' they appropriately call upon all three forms of justice: distributive, corrective and procedural. But, whatever the theoretical route one takes, Tawney's insight remains: social justice addresses inequalities created by social and political organisation. Social justice is about equality.

Disability critique

Many disability scholars, however, are uncomfortable with equality-grounded theories of social justice that attempt to incorporate both aspects of impairments. They remind us of one of the most influential, though usually unstated assumptions of social policy: it is always cheaper, more efficient, and publicly acceptable to provide resources that respond to individual functional deficits, than to modify the physical and social environment in which they live. Not only does the assumption relegate disability policy to the fringes – 'special needs' for people who can't make it in the real world – it also ignores the lessons of the universal-design movement that argue that proactive changes in the physical and social environment are economically efficient and benefit everyone. But the assumption continues to hold the policy sector in its grip, creating a bias in favour of changing the person rather than changing the world. This, the disability critique concludes, further entrenches the true source of social inequality, namely the belief that disabilities are individual deficits that require 'special' services, rather than disadvantages resulting from unjust social arrangements.

The disability critique of mainstream equality theories is undoubtedly sound. When justice theorists turn to disability, there is an immediate shift to impairments, understood as individual deficiencies. We read that justice requires health resources in order to equalise social opportunities (Daniels 1986), or a hypothetical insurance scheme to calculate fair compensation (Dworkin 1981), or resources to equalise positive freedom by raising levels of capability (Sen 1993), or repairing the inequality of marginal utility caused by 'health-related conditions that might be expected to reduce welfare' (Stein 2007: 16). An obsession with personal deficits and comparative well-being of persons with disability may not be demeaning, as Silvers (1994) argues, but it certainly skews the discussion away from social and political organisations and their role in creating the disadvantages of disability, and the feasibility and social and economic advantages of doing so.

A problem

So, is Tawney's insight correct? Does a social commitment to equality not demand that we eliminate (possibly by means of compensation rather than amelioration) inequalities of individual differences, but rather only those inequalities that flow from the operation of social and political organisation? If we recall our gentle interpretative elaboration of Tawney, then we need to add the nuance that the *failure to respond* to needs created by individual differences are also socially created inequalities, a fact that disability scholars should be mindful of should they be tempted to say that impairment is not at all the proper focus of social equality (see again, Shakespeare 2006).

Conceptually, all of this accords perfectly with the interactive model of disability (implicit in the epidemiological models of disability mentioned above): Disability is an outcome of an interaction between attributes of the individual (impairments and functional incapacities) and the entire physical, social, attitudinal, political and culture world in which the individual lives and acts. Impairments and other health problems impact on a person's capacity to participate in life activities; and the individual environment, and response or lack of response to impairment, will also impact on participation. In specific instances, it is not always clear whether the impairment is the major source of the non-participatory outcome, or whether the environment is the primary source. It depends on the facts.

Tawney's insight, the state of the art of equality theorising and the disability critique have all led us back to the interactive understanding of disability, which is arguably our best bet for a workable disability agenda for social justice. But Tawney raises an issue that may limit the effectiveness of this agenda. Why is this agenda about disability alone? How do impairments differ from other disadvantageous individual differences, such as the inability to speak French, the lack of training to repair cars, ignorance of nuclear physics, the absence of musical talent, the lack of the skill of public-speaking – in a word, *non-talents*? If justice and a social commitment to equality require a measured and multi-dimensional response to disability, why not also to the disadvantages linked to non-talents?

Why not, indeed? Both impairments and non-talents are intrinsic differences that are regularly stigmatised and misunderstood, both are 'deficiencies in the individual's capacity to convert external resources into well-being or to press external resources into the service of their chosen ends' (Wasserman 1998: 173), and both interact with the person's broader physical and social environment to create disadvantage. People develop their ambitions and goals in light of both lack of talent and impairment; people cope and adapt to both.

On the face of it, the conceptual similarity between impairments and non-talents seems more like a theoretical curiosity than a practical problem. But no theorist would ever agree that impairments and non-talents are alike in the morally relevant respects. And for good reason. A social policy dedicated to eliminating inequality of all disadvantageous individual differences (skills, talents, abilities, ambitions, life plans) would have devastating, indeed unimaginably dire, consequences. The resources required to eliminate these inequalities would far outstrip the resources available to do so; and in time, the agenda would grind to a halt, as fewer and fewer resources were generated. To avoid this policy black hole, one must clearly distinguish impairments from non-talents. The trick, however, is how to do so.

Distinguishing impairments from non-talents

Approach A: impairments are health problems

Norman Daniels (1986) grants that both impairments and deficits in talent and skill reduce the range of opportunities open to a person. Still, he argues, a person with an impairment has a special claim on society since impairments 'reduce the range of opportunity open to the individual in which he may construct his "plan of life" or conception of the good life' (Daniels 1986: 292). But isn't this true of deficits in talents and skills as well? Daniels responds that impairments are in the domain of health, and the distribution of health-care resources crucially affects a person's access to all good things, and as such is a social justice priority. Justice only requires the equalisation of opportunity for persons with similar skills and talents, not those with different skills and talents.

Daniels' argument for the social priority of health restoration arose as a response to John Rawls' Tawney-like claim that justice does not require society to be held to account for all 'natural inequalities', or even to compensate for them. Society is merely obliged to mitigate natural inequalities by ensuring that social arrangements do not compound or aggravate natural inequalities (Rawls 1971). Arguments by post-Rawlsians like Daniels and Thomas Pogge (Pogge 1989) that health-related inequalities do indeed come under the scope of justice were designed to repair what was thought to be a flaw in Rawlsian justice. The technique used is similar to the interpretative elaboration of Tawney I offered earlier: natural inequalities may not be the proper focus of equality, but a social failure to respond to them in some manner is. The tactic taken by Daniels in particular, however, adds a health rider: equality does not require society to eliminate all natural differences that may affect our opportunities and well-being, only those that are health decrements in normal human functioning.

Predictably, disability scholars flatly reject this approach as it reeks of the medical model of disability, with its exaggerated and prejudicial obsession with 'normal functioning'. Prudent disability scholars do not deny that impairments are health problems that may require health interventions, but they reject playing the 'health card' in the way Daniels does. And they are right to do so, although for a different reason. The health criterion is at best an ambiguous and unpredictable tool for distinguishing impairments from non-talents.

Some skills and talents are themselves functional capacities (running, singing, problem-solving); others causally depend on them (remembering orders as a wait-ress, driving a taxi, pronouncing French words). More generally, all skills and tal-ents depend on functional capacities. That does not mean that, for example, the talent of delivering an entertaining philosophy lecture is itself a 'health ability', merely that it may depend on one's state of health. The fact that skills and talents require functional capacities entails that the health criterion for distinguishing them depends on drawing a line on a causal continuum that is unavoidably arbitrary.

More generally, there are no structural differences between impairments and non-talents that can be grounded in health. We cannot, for example, say that func-tional capacities are simple and atomic while talents are complex and molecular (an impairment in the capacity to learn to read is highly complex, while the talent to whistle two octaves above middle C is simple, but uncommon). Nor could we elaborate on, so to speak, the etiology of impairments and non-talents by arguing that functional capacities are inborn while skills and talents are acquired or devel-oped. Many impairments are acquired and some skills are congenital. The health criterion is a failure.

Yet, the inborn-versus-acquired distinction, even if it fails to operationalise the health domain, does point us towards a common way of distinguishing impair-ments and lacks in talents: functional capacities and their deficits, are part of the person's basic repertoire or endowment, but skill and talents require some effort to develop or acquire, and are to that extent voluntary. This is a very common view, even in the disability community. It is implicit, for example, in the stated rationale of the recently proposed Americans with Disabilities Restoration Act 2007 to the effect that people with disabilities who possess 'the talents, skills, abilities, and desires to participate in society' are precluded from doing so because of discrimination. Granted that in the continuum between 'inborn' and 'acquired', talents seem to be more clearly towards the *inborn* end, while skills lie further in the direction of *acquired*, still the measure being sent is that we are generally not to blame for our impairments, but can be blamed for those non-impairments that require effort to acquire or develop.

Approach B: impairments are not blameworthy

Unfortunately, what might be called the responsibility criterion fails at the outset to draw the line we need: people can be blamed for risky behaviour that leads to injuries causing impairments; and some skills – perfect pitch or gazelle-like gracefulness of movement – may not require development, voluntary or not.

But we should not move on without commenting on the moralistic underpin-nings of this criterion: 'You have only yourself to blame if you did not learn to read; but if you are functionally incapable of learning to read, then you cannot be blamed.' Surely, the claim is, we do not compensate the talent-less, unless it is a medical problem. Perhaps so, but our reason for thinking so has nothing to do with any intrinsic difference, it is a purely moralistic overlay. Wasserman perceptively notes that the health/non-health distinction supplemented by the responsibility criterion is often used as a political device for allocating resources: 'A student who has little talent for math gets lower grades; a student with "dyscalculia" gets tutoring, extra time for exams, or a waiver of math proficiency requirements' (Wasserman 1998: 158). Elsewhere he develops this point, and explores its political and legal ramifications, for the fraught example of alcohol and drug addiction (Wasserman 2004).

But the point here should not be lost. From the perspective of social justice and a commitment to equality, both the health/non-health distinction and the responsibility criteria are morally arbitrary. If we think it just for the student with dyscalculia to get resources and accommodations, then why not do the same favour to the student with bad math grades because of lack of talent, or lack of trying? The consequential personal and social disadvantages will surely be the same for both students. Laziness or lack of motivation need not be labelled 'medical' problems for them to have clear and devastating consequences for the person. If anything, the student who has the ability or talent to learn math, but for complex psychological and sociological reasons does not, may have more need of resources and accommodations than a person with a medically acceptable impairment.

Approach C: talents are positional goods

The example of education suggests another direction we can try. As a resource, education provides people with a competitive edge, one they can exploit to accumulate resources and thereby increase their wealth, social position, and overall well-being. The availability of educational resources is a matter that is within the scope of state action, as is the quality of the educational resources. And availability and quality matter a great deal. A private market in educational resources puts the children of the wealthy at a relative advantage. This means, in the jargon, education is a positional good (Hirsch 1976; Hollis 1984).

A positional good is one whose value to the holder depends on his or her relative position in the distribution of the good. The value of an education, or at least its instrumental value, depends on how much education others possess and who is in competition for the same job or social position. Fair competition – an obvious goal of social justice – mandates a social concern that unfair competitive edges be, if not eliminated, then blunted. In the case of education, this entails social resources to raise the level of education in the public sector to a degree where the competitive edge of a private education is moderated, or eliminated.

One's repertoire of talents and skills – especially those that are marketable – are also positional goods, in the somewhat extended sense that they are amenable to alteration given favourable distribution of relevant positional resources, such as training and education. A fair distribution of talents and skills would mandate social redistribution of those resources so as to bring everyone up to a level of fair competition in the labour market.

Health, some have argued, is an example of a non-positional good, since the value of health to me is independent of the relative level of health of other people. Or as we might say, although health is an instrumental value, it is also an absolute value. Therefore, an inequality of distribution of health care – as is created in a private health-care system – is not problematic from a justice perspective (although efforts to ensure an effective and accessible public system are justifiable to avoid public health problems and other social problems). Hence, chronic decrements of health and functional capacity, or impairments, are non-positional goods.

Here, then, is another version of Tawney's insight: only socially created (or socially allowed) relative differences in advantage are the proper concern of social justice, since positional goods can and should be allocated so as to create fair (that is, equal) competition. Individual differences, such as health differences, are non-positional, so not the proper concern of social justice. Disability, by contrast, is the proper object of social justice, but only to the extent to which the disadvantages of disability can be traced to the operation of social and political organisation (rather than health differences as such).

Although disability scholars might well be tempted by this approach (since it focuses on the social and political causes of disadvantage and neutralises the social significance of impairment), it crumbles on inspection. As Brighouse and Swift (2006) have argued, it is absurd to deny that one's health has relative, competitive value. Its status as a positional good may be latent rather than manifest (Merton 1968), but literature on social determinants of health, while not establishing unambiguous causal connections, has given us plenty of reason to suspect that income and social status inequality are associated with, and perpetuated by, health inequality (e.g. Wilkinson 1996). This evidence overwhelming supports the policy of treating health care resources as positional goods.

Approach D: ignoring the difference is dangerous

Conceptually distinguishing impairments from non-talents may not be a fruitful endeavour; certainly most theorists who rely on the distinction have put little effort into being careful about the distinction. Perhaps they feel that the distinction is too obvious to need conceptual clarity. More likely, as I begun this discussion by noting, they believe that unless a distinction is made, social chaos, of the 'floodgates' variety, would ensue. If we do not distinguish impairments from non-talents, or disabilities from the disadvantages of lack of skill or talent, they argue, then a social commitment to equality will lead to massive, oppressive and politically unacceptable, redistribution of resources. The end result would be the *bête noire* of all egalitarians: levelling down.

A powerful objection to welfare and resource egalitarians of every shape and colour is that without a redistributive threshold limit (such as relative marginal utility or priority to the worse off) the egalitarian impulse would reduce the welfare or resources of those better-off to a level matching those who are worse off in order to achieve equality (Parfit 2000; Stein 2006; Temkin 2000). A few critics go so far as to insist that levelling down is an inevitable result of *any* account of social equality (Frankfurt 1987). The concern is that egalitarians, if left to their own devices, would perversely opt for an equally divided pie of welfare or resources rather than an unequally divided pie in which the smallest slice is bigger than what is delivered by equal division. Egalitarians, it is argued, fixate on the relative position and ignore the absolute position of the worse off.

If this is a genuine challenge to egalitarianism, our question is: would it make any difference if egalitarianism applied only to impairments and not non-talents? The answer is not at all, especially if, as we saw, it is plausible to character- ise health as a positional good. Once again, utilitarians have insisted that non- utilitarian egalitarian redistributive policy for impairments alone would demand that welfare or resources be distributed away from those with no or – more real- istically – with only minor impairments to the benefit of those with the most or the most severe impairments. Others go much further and repeat Robert Nozick's paranoid fantasy (which he later disowned) of the state requiring redistribution of body parts or blinding the sighted in order to achieve true equality (Nozick 1974; Temkin 2000).

At this point, we might lose faith with egalitarianism itself and, like many phi- losophers in recent years, follow Derek Parfit's move (Parfit 2000) towards 'pri- oritarian' accounts that assign redistributive priority to the 'worst off' in society and abandon the prospect of an overall reduction of inequality. Alternatively, we might be attracted to a utilitarian approach, say, the powerful version recently described by Mark Stein (Stein 2006), and opt for a distributive policy under the firm control of a criterion of marginal utility.

If we are so tempted, we would not have made much progress on our problem. Neither prioritarians nor utilitarians have managed to distinguish impairments from non-talents in a conceptually rigorous and non-ad hoc fashion. Prioritarians are more concerned in dealing with the thorny problem of devising a non-ques- tion-begging characterisation of who in society is 'worst off', while for their part, utilitarians would be hard pressed to distinguish impairments from non-talents on the basis of any workable definition of welfare or utility. If we are looking for help in distinguishing impairments from non-talents, we cannot look here.

Approach E: ignore the difference anyway

Some egalitarians seem to get around our problem by offering accounts suffi- ciently vague about the sources of disadvantageous inequality as to apply to both impairments and non-talents. For example, Ronald Dworkin's hypothetical insur- ance scheme is designed to deal indifferently with the 'brute bad luck' of impair- ments, limited or non-existent talents, and other examples of inadequate internal resources. The hypothetical insurance scheme works like this: people ignorant of their life plans are asked what they would be willing to pay by way of insurance were they to acquire these disadvantages, and when consensus on this figure is reached, it would, by definition, constitute fair compensation of the inadequacy (Dworkin 1981).

A very different proposal by Amartya Sen (1993) characterises 'capabilities' as those things and activities that people have a realistic choice over, the sum total of which constitutes the person's range of positive freedom. Capabilities, so defined, are both internal and external resources, so the egalitarian programme would direct social resources to remove external and internal barriers. Non-talents as well as impairments would seem to qualify as internal functional decrements for Sen.

There is much that can be said about both of these theories, but for our discussion it is relevant to note that neither successfully confronts the floodgates worry of burdensome redistribution. Sen seems to escape this challenge by keeping his discussion abstract, to such an extent that some have argued that if Sen's account were ever applied in practice, it would only work if it transformed itself into a version of welfare utilitarianism in order to set limits to distribution (Stein 2006). Against Dworkin, it needs only be said that he ignores Tawney's insight that justice demands, not merely compensation for inadequate internal resources, but the removal of inequality caused by social and political organisation. When removal is impossible, or impossibly costly, then compensation is a good, second-best, solution. But people with disabilities have a strong moral claim to remove external barriers and eliminate stigma and discrimination, and this claim is utterly ignored by the insurance approach.

Approach F: deal with both in terms of a distributive threshold

Perhaps both impairments and non-talents can be handled in a theory of equality if the goal of redistribution is not the elimination of inequality, but the elimination of a level of inequality that can be independently argued to be at the moral core of equality and so really matter to us. The idea here is to tame justice of distribution by reversing Tawney's approach and subsuming it under procedural justice. Amy Gutmann, for example, argues that justice only demands that the procedural goal of 'democratic equality' be secured. Democratic equality is secured when economic and social redistribution eliminates those (but only those) disparities that threaten to undermine participation in social and political roles essential in a democratic organisation (Gutmann 1987). Using the example of education, she argues that justice requires educational resource distribution sufficient to provide all children with abilities required to participate in the democratic process. Redistribution would be focused on both non-talents and impairments alike (so the distinction would no longer matter), but only insofar as their redress would facilitate democratic equality.

Elizabeth Anderson (1999) adds further detail to democratic equality. Following Iris Marion Young (1990), she argues that egalitarianism has traditionally set its sights in opposition to unequal social relations – in the form of marginalisation, status hierarchy, domination, exploitation and cultural imperialism – not, as the current debate has it, against differences in 'fortune and brute luck'. At most, she insists, justice requires that everyone possess those Senian capabilities that are required to live as equal citizens in a democratic society. And that is enough for our moral intuitions.

Since the account depends on the plausibility of this point, it is fair to ask of Anderson how she would characterise these essential, threshold capabilities.

Anderson provides us with three dimensions of capability required for equal democratic citizenship, and the resources required for each dimension:

1. *to be capable of functioning as a human being:* 'effective access to the means of sustaining one's biological existence – food, shelter, clothing, medical care – and access to the basic conditions of human agency – knowledge of one's circumstances and options, the ability to deliberate about means and ends, the psychological conditions of autonomy, including the self-confidence to think and judge for oneself, freedom of thought and movement.'
2. *to be capable of functioning as a participant in a system of cooperative production:* 'effective access to the means of production, access to the education needed to develop one's talents, freedom of occupational choice, the right to make contracts and enter into cooperative agreements with others, the right to receive fair value for one's labour, and recognition by others of one's productive contributions.'
3. *to be capable of functioning as a citizen of a democratic state:* 'effective access to rights to political participation, such as freedom of speech and the franchise, and also effective access to the goods and relationships of civil society (e.g. freedom of association, access to public spaces and services, freedom to form relationships, privacy).'

(Anderson 1999: 318–19)

Anderson makes much of the fact that democratic equality avoids the levelling-down objection by, in effect, heeding Tawney's insight that it is not 'natural diversity' that needs to be tamed, but socially created oppressive hierarchies: 'Instead of lamenting the human diversity of talents and trying to make up for what is represented as innate deficiencies in talent, democratic equality offers a way of conceiving and harnessing human diversity as that it benefits everyone' (ibid.: 336). She also insists that democratic equality need not require resource redistribution as much as changing norms and the structure of public goods. Finally, she echoes disability activists who argue that providing resources to compensate for impairments as individual deficiencies is demeaning.

Unfortunately, as Wasserman has noted (1998), Anderson paradoxically has set the threshold for equality both too low and too high. As an account of procedural rather than distributive justice, she strives to ensure equal rights and freedoms, equal access and fair procedures, consistent with democratic membership. But by thus ignoring both welfare and resource inequalities, the value of these procedures will always be threatened by those who can rely on their talents and wealth to turn them to their own advantage. In effect, procedural rights in a context of distributional *inequality of resources* become positional goods open to competition – freedoms and rights that can be bought and sold. Her standard of equality, in short, is far too feeble. On the other hand, for individuals with substantial health needs, or severe cognitive and emotional impairments, her 'capacity to be a human being', and especially to secure the 'basic conditions of human agency', may well be a unreachable threshold or else hugely costly in resources.

Disability as a demographic: entrenching the difference

But there is something even more troubling about the project of democratic equality. Far from ignoring the difference between impairments and non-talents, democratic equality entrenches the distinction in a manner that greatly increases the social disadvantages of non-talents. The grounding purpose of democratic equality is to preserve the freedom of the market and talent meritocracy. Oppressive and discriminatory hierarchies based on impairments can be eliminated by means of access to rights and freedoms. But hierarchies based on talent will remain, since any attempt to 'equalise fortune' will require oppressive state action. It is essential to democratic equality that everyone has the freedom to develop their talents and skills, and reap the benefits thereof. Meritocracy and economic inequality are social consequences of that freedom, given a natural diversity of distribution of talent.

It is fair to ask whether it is enough to provide for impairment needs and eliminate the discriminatory disadvantages of disability. To be sure, a person with a disability may have a talent (or the ability to develop one) but has been prevented from doing so by discrimination. So too, ameliorating the impact of impairments may facilitate the development of new skills. Yet, it is very naïve to think that social justice for persons with impairments will create for each individual *new talents or skills* that were not already there. If we assume, as seems reasonable, that special talents and skills – those with high competitive value in the free market – are distributed randomly between persons with impairments and those without, then at best Anderson's democratic equality will have the outcome of including, on a fair and equal basis, individuals with impairments into the competitive meritocracy.

Obviously, this is not a minor social achievement. But it is also a surprisingly limited one. Suppose we characterise the ideal of a procedurally fair and equal society as one in which purely demographic distinctions do not skew the random distribution of talents and skills. That is, the prevalence of talent and skill in some domain, across race, gender, sexual orientation, ethnic background, and so on, ought to be more or less the same. And this cut across the impairment divide. As talents and skills play out in a free market, the diversity of talents and skills will be reflected in the distribution of wealth, resources, and social position. There will be winners and losers, rich and poor. Anderson's democratic equality, if achievable, would ensure that, directly proportional to their representation in the overall population, there will be an equal number of rich men as rich women, rich blacks as whites, and rich people with and without impairments. Likewise for the poor. In the procedural just democratic state, impairment is fully integrated into meritocracy. Or to use a slightly different idiom, disability will be *universalised and mainstreamed*, an explicit goal of many disability activists (see an early statement by Zola 1989).

It may be that fully integrating people with impairments into hierarchies of welfare and social position supported by talent meritocracy is the proper and ultimate objective of social justice with respect to disability. It would certainly be a vast improvement on the current situation in which people with impairments are either completely sidelined from participation in social institutions, or so greatly disadvantaged by lack of accommodation and discrimination as not in any sense to enjoy full and complete participation in society. Arguably, our comfort level for this goal of social equality should depend on how severe the resulting meritocracy is, and in particular the distance, in terms of welfare, between the rich and the poor. Is it really a goal worth striving for to have proportionally equal number of people with impairments starving in the streets as people without impairments? But, be that as it may, as should be obvious, the democratic equality approach depends entirely on a clear and operational distinction between impairments and the non-talents. We have come full circle.

Conclusion: where does this leave us?

There are two fundamental approaches to the conceptualisation of disability: the categorical (dichotomous) and the continuous. Social policy demands the categorical approach, since for all disability programming one must be able to define the target population. An individual either qualifies as disabled, or does not. It cannot be a matter of degree. (Continuous eligibility is theoretically possible, but complex and expensive, and at any rate has not been tried in practice.) Yet, conceptually and scientifically, impairment is a continuous phenomenon, a matter of more or less.

If we turn to the epidemiological model of functioning and disability found in WHO's ICF, bodily functioning and structure are classified by domain – mental, sensory, voice, functions of the cardiovascular, respiratory, digestive, genitourinary, reproductive systems, neuromusculoskeletal, and skin – and each of these is further divided into more and more detailed sub-domains. Impairment can occur in any of these domains, to any degree from severe to mild. An individual may have impairments in one or several domains at the same time, to one or another degree. (Indeed, every human being has some degree of impairment in some domain or other.) The variety of impairment is therefore immense. On top of that, the full and complete lived experience of having impairments (that is, being disabled) is also highly variable, for personal and social and cultural environmental reasons.

So, how do we answer questions about who is disabled or the prevalence of disability in a country or region? As a multi-domain, multi-dimensional, interactive and continuous phenomenon (as it is characterised in the ICF), we must specify which impairment domains qualify, to which degree of severity. Different prevalence answers flow from different decisions. If we are interested in any impairment domain, to any degree of severity, then prevalence is roughly universal – a conclusion of no use to policy-makers whatsoever. If we restrict our scope to specific domains and severity levels, then our prevalence results will differ accordingly. But these decisions cannot be made conceptually or scientifically; they are political. The scientific approach, in a word, does not solve the problem the policy analyst needs to solve.

Traditionally, disability prevalence figures have been based on categorical and dichotomous impairment data: what is counted is the number of people who are blind, deaf, missing limbs, paralysed, or cognitively impaired. Often, people with specified diseases or congenital deformations were added to expand the numbers. The categories selected were politically negotiable, although people with disabilities rarely if ever were asked to participate in the negotiations. This is what it means to treat the disability category as a demographic. With agreed prevalence data, policies and programmes can be motivated, devised, costed, and monitored.

In practice, in short, the distinction between impairments and non-talents is implicitly, or covertly, made on political and economic grounds. There is no scientific or conceptual ground for the distinction.

To make matters more difficult, not infrequently the impairment continuum overlaps (or is coincident with) the talent continuum. That is, some impairments are (or might as well be) non-talents, whereas the absence of an impairment is (or might as well be) a talent. To take just one example, if one is out-going, self-confident and socially aggressive, one is in possession of competitively useful talents (or perhaps, components of talents). By contrast, if one has traits at the other end of the continuum, and is shy and timid, one has potentially socially disadvantageous non-talents. As a rule, people fall on a continuum in this domain, from highly aggressive and reckless to obsessively shy ('social anxiety'). Since both extremes have adverse consequences for people (or are linked symptomatically to mental or emotional disorders) both extremes are thought to be impairments. Only the middle ground is clearly the absence of an impairment. But where precisely, on the edges of that middle ground, an impairment shades off into a lack of talent or a talent is impossible to tell, both because we do not typically make such finely granular distinctions, and because cultural and socially considerations will determine that the line should be drawn in very different places. At the end of the day, if there is need to make the distinction, we will; where there is no need to do so, we will not.

Where does this leave us? Tawney's insight was that differences between people – the fact that some are shy and others self-confident – are not differences that a social commitment to equality should be concerned about. But when these, or other differences, are made important by our social and political organisation (or when they are a product of our institutions), then our concern for equality is engaged. There are historical and sociological reasons why some impairments, at some level of severity, are individual differences that matter medically and socially. For other historical and sociological reasons, some non-talents, even when in the same domain and along the same continuum of functioning as impairments, do not matter medically or socially. If you are so shy you can't hold a job or form meaningful relationships, that's your problem. But if you are so shy that you have 'social anxiety', that is not your problem. Where this line is drawn, is, apparently, for the fates to decide.

Bibliography

Altman, B. R. (2001) 'Disability Definitions, Models, Classification Schemes, and Applications', in G. Albrecht, K. Seelman and M. Bury (eds), *Handbook of Disability Studies*, Thousand Oaks, CA: Sage.

Amundson, R. (1992) 'Disability, Handicap, and the Environment', *Journal of Social Philosophy*, 23: 105–18.

Anderson, E. (1999) 'What Is the Point of Equality?', *Ethics*, 109: 287–337.

Bagenstos, S. R. (2000) 'Subordination, Stigma, and "Disability"', *Virginia Law Review*, 86: 397–534.

—— (2003) 'The Americans with Disabilities Act as Welfare Reform', *Williams and Mary Law Journal*, 44: 1–89.

Bickenbach, J. (1993) *Physical Disability and Social Policy*, Toronto: University of Toronto Press.

Brighouse, H. and Swift, A. (2006) 'Equality, Priority, and Positional Goods', *Ethics*, 116: 471–95.

Daniels, N. (1986) 'Justice and Health Care', in D. Van DeVeer and T. Regan (eds), *Health Care Ethics: An Introduction*, Philadelphia, PA: Temple University Press.

Dworkin, R. (1981) 'What Is Equality? Part 2: Equality of Resources', *Philosophy and Public Affairs*, 10: 283–345.

Fougeyrollas, P. (1995) 'Documenting Environmental Factors for Preventing the Handicap Creation Process', *Disability and Rehabilitation*, 17: 83–102.

Frankfurt, H. G. (1987) 'Equality as a Moral Ideal', *Ethics*, 98: 21–43.

Gutmann, A. (1987) *Democratic Education*, Princeton, NJ: Princeton University Press.

Hahn, H. (1988) 'The Politics of Physical Differences: Disability and Discrimination', *Journal of Social Issues*, 44: 43–68.

Hirsch, F. (1976) *Social Limits to Growth*, Cambridge, MA: Harvard University Press.

Hollis, M. (1984) 'Education as a Positional Good', *Journal of Philosophy of Education*, 22: 235–44.

Merton, R. K. (1968) *Social Theory and Social Structure*, Glencoe, IL: Free Press.

Nagi, S. Z. (1965) 'Some Conceptual Issues in Disability and Rehabilitation', in M. B. Sussman (ed.), *Sociology and Rehabilitation*, Washington, DC: American Sociological Association.

Nozick, R. (1974) *Anarchy, State and Utopia*, New York: Basic Books.

Nussbaum, M. (1992) 'Human Functioning and Social Justice: A Defense of Aristotelian Essentialism', *Political Theory*, 20: 202–46.

Oliver, M. (1986) 'Social Policy and Disability: Some Theoretical Issues', *Disability, Handicap and Society*, 1: 5–17.

Parfit, D. (2000) 'Equality and Priority', in M. Clayton and A. Williams (eds), *The Ideal of Equality*, Basingstoke: Palgrave Macmillan.

Pogge, T. W. (1989) *Realising Rawls*, Ithaca, NY: Cornell University Press.

Rawls, J. (1971) *A Theory of Justice*, Cambridge, MA: Harvard University Press.

Saflios-Rothschild, C. (1970) *The Sociology and Social Psychology of Disability and Rehabilitation*, New York: Random House.

Sen, A. (1980) 'Equality of What?', in S. McMurrin (ed.), *Tanner Lectures on Human Values*, Salt Lake City, UT: University of Utah Press.

—— (1993) 'Capability and Well-Being', in M. Nussbaum and A. Sen (eds), *The Quality of Life*, Oxford: Clarendon Press.

Shakespeare, T. (2006) *Disability Rights and Wrongs*, London: Routledge.

Silvers, A. (1994) '"Defective" Agents: Equality, Difference and the Tyranny of the Normal', *Journal of Social Philosophy*, 25th Anniversary Special Issue: 154–75.

Stein, M. S. (2003) 'The Law and Economics of Disability Accommodations', *Duke Law Journal*, 53: 79–192.

—— (2006) *Distributive Justice and Disability: Utilitarianism against Egalitarianism*, New Haven, CT: Yale University Press.

Tawney, R. H. (1931) *Equality*, London: Allen and Unwin.

Temkin, L. (2000) 'Equality, Priority and the Levelling Down Objection', in M. Clayton and A. Williams (eds), *The Ideal of Equality*, Basingstoke: Palgrave Macmillan.

Union of the Physically Impaired Against Segregation (UPIAS) (1976) *Fundamental Principles of Disability*, London: UPIAS.

Wasserman, D. (1996) 'Some Moral Issues in the Correction of Impairments', *Journal of Social Philosophy*, 27: 128–45.

—— (1998) 'Distributive Justice', in A. Silvers, D. Wasserman and M. B. Mahowald (eds), *Disability, Difference, Discrimination*, Lanham, MD: Rowman and Littlefield.

—— (2004) 'Addiction and Disability: Moral and Policy Issues', *Substance Use and Misuse*, 39: 461–88.

Wilkinson, R. (1996) *Unhealthy Societies: The Afflictions of Inequality*, London: Routledge.

Williams, G. (2001) 'Theorising Disability', in G. Albrecht, K. Seelman and M. Bury (eds), *Handbook of Disability Studies*, Thousand Oaks, CA: Sage Publications.

World Health Organisation (2001) *International Classification of Functioning, Disability and Health (ICF)*, Geneva: WHO.

Wright, B. (1983) *Physical Disability: A Psychosocial Approach*, 2nd edn, New York: Harper and Row.

Young, I. M. (1990) *Justice and the Politics of Difference*, Princeton, NJ: Princeton University Press.

Zola, I. K. (1989) 'Toward the Necessary Universalising of a Disability Policy', *The Millbank Quarterly*, 67: 401–28.

8 Gender, disability and personal identity

Moral and political problems in community thinking

Tuija Takala

The notion of 'community' plays a central role in disability studies (Longmore 2003: 222–3). While positive values such as solidarity, altruism and together-ness are often linked with the idea of community, other issues also arise, such as exclusion, division and separation (Takala and Häyry 2004: 276). In this chapter I examine the implications of using *community* as the main focus point when discussing some ethical issues related to disability. The limits of the usefulness of this concept are studied, and I will show how reliance on communal consider-ations alone might lead to detrimental consequences. I do not claim that commu-nity thinking should be totally disregarded, nor that community values should be altogether dismissed. I will, however, argue that there are limits to what notions of community can do for us, and that perhaps other considerations should be taken into account. In this chapter, I will be looking at disabled people as a group that is judged against the 'gold standard' of our societies, at the bodily aspects of such classifications, at the pros and cons of oppressed groups uniting together, and at the notion of the victim position. I will conclude by suggesting that because of the untoward consequences of classifying people, we should perhaps not label and categorise human beings, when and if this is possible.

I myself am not disabled and hence cannot speak from a personal perspective with regard to this. I am, however, a member of another group which, similar to disabled people, has been and continues to be subject to oppression, a group whose membership is designated based on bodily features, a group which has gained much political power by uniting, and a group that continues to provide strength to many of its members: I am a woman. My somewhat bold hypoth-esis in this chapter is that in many important senses, the experiences of being a woman and being disabled are comparable. This, I hope, will add a lived element to my analysis concerning the notion of community. There are further similarities between the two groups: both of them have political and theoretical dimensions which tend to overlap. In this chapter, I use the word 'oppression' to mean every-day practices, not necessarily motivated by maleficent intentions, but those which place people in certain groups with positions where they are disadvantaged and suffer from injustice (Young 2006: 4).

Other people classify us and we classify others. We are Asians, Europeans, men, women, homosexual, heterosexual, working class, middle class, disabled, athletes, academics, drunkards, environmentalists, bohemians, artists, activists, parents, teachers, policemen, soldiers, unemployed, politicians, civil servants, doctors, humanists, Catholics, Buddhists, atheists, hippies, yuppies, nerds, technocrats, and so on. The list is endless. By labelling people, we allow much of our everyday lives to be based on stereotypical categories. To some extent this helps us to get by without having to intimately know all the people we come in contact with: if a person is 'such and such', then I can and should treat her in a particular manner. We expect people to live more or less in accordance with their respective roles. Most of us, however, I would hope, consider people close to us as individuals rather than representatives of certain groups.

Against the gold standard

Women and disabled people, like many other oppressed groups in our societies, are constantly placed in a position of the 'other' when it comes to their achievements. We live in an age where an able-bodied white (usually Christian) heterosexual man is the gold standard in our societies. Say the talk is about 'the leading scientist', 'the best painter' or 'the greatest composer', in all of these phrases the general expectation seems to be that the person belongs to the above-mentioned group. However, if the person happens to be, say, a woman, disabled, black or a Muslim, this characteristic will be mentioned fairly quickly when his or her achievements are discussed. But, when people fit the gold standard, their sex, physical condition, religion or ethnic origin will often not be mentioned: that was only what was to be expected anyway, since 'he' is the norm as far as achievements go. For the rest of us, it is, at its best, a 'damn good for a woman'[1] world.

The gold-standard thinking can also be seen as an expression of non-maleficent oppression. Often, people with disabilities, and women alike, choose to emphasise their otherness when they have achieved something of importance. The hope is to break with the typical classifications by showing that also a woman or a disabled person is able to achieve something in a gold standard-dominated area. The problem is that this does little to challenge the gold standard. It might prove that there are some exceptions, but the standard itself remains untouched. The labels assigned to others are a forceful way of upholding existing power structures (Sparti 2001: 336–9). Those who need not to be labelled are the ones in whose interests it is to continue labelling others and to maintain the status quo: they are the ones with power.

Bodily features cause bodily positions of disadvantage

Being discriminated against and suffering oppression are not only problems for women or for disabled people. Ethnic origin, nationality, sexual orientation, social class and religion are among other common bases for discrimination. It was actually only a century ago that race and gender were thought to be literally disabling factors by the scientific community (Amundson 2005: 122). I would, however, argue that unlike, say, ethnic origin which is also sometimes a visible bodily feature that can put people in a position of disadvantage, it is only disabled people and women who share bodily features that are both used in their classification and put them in a position of *bodily* disadvantage. Obviously, the differences between the various impairments behind disability vary considerably, but for argument's sake, let us think here of conditions that lead to slightly limited opportunities only. It is with these that some of the experiences of disabled people can be seen as analogous to those encountered by women.

As a woman, I am for a large part of my life restricted in my activities (as opposed to my male counterparts) due to my menstrual cycle. If I am thinking of going on hiking trips, spending time in primitive lodgings, swimming or engaging in sport activities, the time of the month when these events happen will have a considerable effect as to the ease or difficulty with which I can participate. For many women, the monthly cycle also brings not-insignificant back and stomach pains, and for some, their psychological states are greatly affected as well. In terms of my sexual relationships, in each close encounter with a fertile male I put myself in the risk of grave intrusion of my bodily integrity, either in terms of pregnancy or of an abortion. This is a burden that no male has to carry. And once my age of fertility ends, I will suffer a variety of problems from hot and cold waves to sleeplessness. Furthermore, to be able to live with the symptoms, I may require medication that is dangerous to my health.

Disability scholars often write about the unease that disabled people feel when the able-bodied discuss disability as an option worse than death (Parens and Asch 1999: 236). Not having been disabled myself, I am not sure whether I can completely understand how it must feel that views such as this are aired so openly, and often without shame.

Based on the hypothesis of this chapter, that the experiences of disabled people and women have some similarities, I have very informally asked some of my male acquaintances about their views on gender and disability. When presented with the question 'If you had the choice between waking up the next morning (a) paralysed from the waist down, (b) with a woman's body (much like your previous one, but with less bodily hair, breasts, and female sex organs instead of a penis), or (c) not waking up at all' the responses have been, to say the least, interesting.

For most of them, finding out that they were women was at least as bad as being paralysed from the waist down, and for everyone, not waking up at all was an option definitely worth considering. When I formulated the options in more realistic ways, by replacing option (b) with option (b1), 'and were told you are actually biologically female, but due to the fact that at birth unusually large labia and some other genital ambiguities were found, surgery was performed to make you look like boys (and that the pills that you have been taking since puberty are not actually vitamins but hormones)',[2] they were slightly less certain about the options. What they seemed most interested in was whether they could keep on 'being' men, or would their femininity begin to show? Their biology did not seem to worry them as much as other people's perception of it did. This change of heart seems to indicate that if it happened to them, being biologically female would not significantly alter their view of themselves, but that they could not trust others to feel the same way. To me, this speaks volumes about related-power structures.

Discrimination unites

With disabled people, as with women, it was oppression from the outside that caused these groups to unite thus creating the 'disabled community' and the 'women's community'. Two disabled persons might have nothing else in common beyond the fact that they are both oppressed because of the label assigned to them: disabled. Similarly, there are women with very different beliefs, values and agendas, but what unites them is the fact that they are met with differential treatment because they are women.

The disability-rights movement and the women's-rights movement have both achieved significant improvements in the ways in which the representatives of these groups are treated in modern societies. The benefits for individuals as members of these groups have been considerable. Women and disabled people are, at least on paper, considered equal citizens, and discrimination based on gender or disability is unlawful, for example, in the job market. Both groups are compensated for the social structures that have placed them in positions of disadvantage. The needs of disabled people are increasingly met, for example, by the educational system, which provides various aids for disabled students to allow them to partake in studies at all levels. Women's roles as main carers for children are compensated by maternity leave, and this is also taken into account as a mediating factor, for instance, when years of job experience are counted.

From external oppression to internal and external oppression

While a united voice gave members of these groups more political power and contributed to change, it came with a price. In order for there to be a united voice, there needs to be unity and shared objectives. But for groups that became united because of a common enemy, further goals shared by all members can be hard to come by. People became 'women' or 'disabled' because these were the classifications used. For sure, many women's lives are, as opposed to men's lives, to varying degrees, shaped by getting pregnant, giving birth, breast-feeding and nurturing children, but this is not true of all women. Furthermore, arguably, women are more prone to thinking about ethics in relational terms (Gilligan 1982), but there are also many women who give more weight to justice considerations (Richards 1982). And while women might be statistically more likely to be linguistically talented and physically weaker than their male counterparts, there are men who are linguistically more talented than the average woman as well as men who are weaker than most females. Whether we are looking at biologically guided social roles, modes of thinking, or various abilities, there is very little evidence to suggest that all women would fit a role that is specific to women only. When talking about disabled people, one could argue that the variations are even greater. In what sense would a congenitally deaf person, someone with a moderate-to-severe learning disorder, and a teenager paralysed after a car accident form a unified group through which each of these individuals would primarily define themselves?

One could argue that the categories 'woman' and 'disabled' are to a large degree social constructions. These categories gained their importance because of the social meanings attached to them. This is not to say that there is no biological difference between men, women and those with ambiguous biological sex, or that there is no bodily impairment contributing to most disabilities. What I am saying here is that the moral and political importance of the categories 'woman' or 'disabled' is primarily linked to their socially constructed meanings. And herein lays one of the anomalies of the disability-rights movement and of the women's-rights movement. Much of the oppression felt by those labelled 'disabled' or 'woman' follows from the fact that these individuals have been categorised as members of these groups, yet the individuals thus classified need to unite with others with similar fates to gain the political power to fight their oppression. However, by uniting, they also contribute to the ends of their oppressors, by re-affirming the justifiability of the original classification (bat Tzedek 2005: 252). This is sometimes known as the 'ghetto effect'. To reiterate, although in many ways the disability-rights movement and the women's-rights movements have accomplished a great deal, if one looks at the matter from another perspective, I would contend that in striving to fight the external oppression they have actually made it stronger.

But, could there be something to the classifications, and should there be? Do disabled people as a group or women as a group share something which should be celebrated? Is there more to their unity than a common enemy? The apparent lack of common goals and shared identity has posed serious problems to the politically motivated women's-rights movement and the disability-rights movement (and to their theoretical counterparts). One answer to the problem has been to nurture community feeling within the group. Many disability activists have found it important to create and strengthen the idea that there is a separate disability culture (Swain and French 2000). The catch in this line of thinking is that while disability is viewed as a social construct and social oppression (a 'bad thing'), it is at the same time expected that one defines oneself as disabled ('good' identity building). Within 'women's community', similar thinking manifests itself in views where women are marginalised because of male dominance ('the socially constructed woman'), while simultaneously being asked to build their identities on their womanhood (bat Tzedek 2005: 256). Depending on which brand of feminism one subscribes to, the tension between these standpoints varies (Hackett and Haslanger 2006).

I have never belonged to any women's network or association (although I have been to one or two meetings), because I have never understood why the fact that all those participating are women would add anything to the experience, or why others should be excluded because they are not women. Let me discuss this more concretely. If there is an Iris Murdoch reading group, I would think everyone interested in her writings should contribute. If someone, for some reason, wishes to discuss Iris Murdoch from the viewpoint of people who, for example, have experienced biological motherhood, I suppose that could be used as an inclusion criterion, but it would not include all women. If someone wants to discuss Murdoch in a non-hostile and friendly setting, I am doubtful as to whether the exclusion of one sex would produce the expected results. There are hostile men and there are hostile women, just as there are warm and caring men and warm and caring women. The fact that someone represents a particular gender is no guarantee as to what the person is like. If I take part in a voluntary activity, I would like others participating to also have an interest in that activity. If it so happens that for a particular group at a particular time, only members of one gender happen to participate, that is of course okay, but I do not see how this could be used as an argument to exclude people of a different gender from taking part later on. By excluding people based on classifications that, at the most, have statistical relevance, is not only discrimination, but might also result in important contributions not being heard. I, for one, see no value in upholding such practices.

The creation of women's culture and the disability culture has produced a new kind of oppression to those labelled 'disabled' or 'woman'. While a unified group speaks in a louder voice, the need for unity does not allow for individualised views, since those would threaten or fragment the community and would thus make the group politically weaker (see Shakespeare 2006). In terms of the well-being of the people who are oppressed because they have been labelled as members of a particular group, it seems that they cannot win. Without a community they are weak and vulnerable, but with the community, there is a danger of being forced to adopt the views of the group. Moreover, arguably, by emphasising the distinctive nature of the group, the members of the group can experience and even invite further marginalisation.

The victim position

Identifying with other people with similar experiences and views has, of course, also its benefits. From a psychological point of view, shared hardships are easier to understand and live with. Belonging to a community that values me as a woman (or as a disabled person) can help me to build the self-esteem that has been damaged by the perceptions and treatments that I, as a woman (or as a disabled person), have received from others. Everyone needs to feel loved and valued. Kinship, solidarity and togetherness are examples of the clear positive effects that strong community commitments can bring to individuals' lives.

On a more cynical note, it is sometimes argued that identifying with an oppressed group allows people to adopt a 'victim position' whereby all the difficulties encountered in life can be explained by being 'a woman' or 'disabled', etc, and hence oppressed. If I did not get a particular job, it could not have been my poor interview-performance or lack of relevant experience, but rather because I was a woman. If this outlook on life is internalised to a greater degree, it allows me to stop trying altogether: no matter what I do, I will not be successful, so I might as well give up.

Talking about the victim position is, however, dangerous. While it seems clear that there are people who have adopted the victim position (more or less consciously) because it has made their lives easier, this does not mean that discrimination does not happen. Sometimes, perhaps more often than not, people do not get what they deserve simply because of the way they have been classified. It should be acknowledged that recognising the phenomenon of victim position and understanding its psychological appeal does not mean that there are no actual victims.

From the viewpoint of disability- or women's-rights activists, the victim position is a two-edged sword. Since it was oppression that brought disabled people (and women) together in the first place and since it is the continuous oppression that, at least partly, keeps them together, everyone within these groups must, to a degree, agree that they are in a position of victims. The problems, however, arise when someone from these groups succeeds beyond what is expected of a woman or of a disabled person as this seems to undermine the victimhood analysis. Too often, the success is met by hostility and by the group disowning the person who makes it (Shakespeare 2006: 80), rather than joining in to celebrate the triumph of one of its members. It is thought that achievements are only possible if one sells out one's true identity. We have all heard people calling Margaret Thatcher 'a man in a skirt', mirrored by similar comments by men and women alike where women in high places in large corporations are described as cold and calculating. The logic is simple enough: we are oppressed by the structures of the male-run and able-bodied dominated society, and to achieve anything huge in that world can only mean that one has adopted the rules of the oppressive forces and hence forfeited one's own kind. This, to me, looks like vicious circle or a 'Catch-22'. On the one hand, fighting the oppression is the only clear common goal, but on the other hand, if an individual succeeds, this means that the person in question has sold out.

Similar questions are sometimes tackled with the concept 'internalised oppression' (Meyers 2002: 3–29). Here the focus is not on the victim, but on those who have willingly or unwittingly accepted the unfair rules of an oppressive society. Again, depending on one's views about what is wrong with existing social structures and why, the seriousness of this accusation, when made, will vary considerably.

Concluding thoughts

After the somewhat discouraging conclusions drawn in this chapter, I should emphasise that I do not think that people should not unite for political or other purposes. We are social animals, and we define ourselves through our communities and the company we keep. Furthermore, I have no doubt that our communities are important sources of well-being and strength, as well as providers of political power. Shared experiences and common goals are necessary in striving for a better life, and we all want to feel a sense of belonging. Within the political arena, it is obvious that to get the voices of minorities and the oppressed heard, collaborations are important and probably necessary. Women and disabled people are good examples of people who have benefited greatly from the group efforts of the political activists.

One of the largest problems with identity politics seems to be that too often it is assumed that we belong to one community only, and that only through that one community do we define ourselves, our values and life projects. While this is in the interests of those who hold the power (keeping people in their boxes makes them easier to control), it is not obviously true. We are members of numerous communities, and these carry significance to our being that varies from time to time (Glover 1988: 200–2). In a Manchester football derby, when City score against United, and immediately after, I might feel a strong sense of togetherness with all the City fans, while at most other times I would have very little in common with most other City supporters. And when, say, people of my nationality or gender are being bullied or joked about, I am likely to feel that I am somehow personally under attack also, while at other times I may not pay much attention to issues of nationality or gender.

Within gender studies and disability studies alike, there has long been recognition of the fact that the one-dimensional classifications are inadequate (Zinn and Dill 2005: 19–25). Often people belong to a number of communities, which, if one only allows for stereotypical readings, assign them to incompatible roles. Also, sometimes the political agenda of a group only seems to acknowledge the needs of some of its sub-groups. For instance, black women often feel that neither the women's community nor the black community addresses their issues (Grillo 2006: 31).

There is an important difference in my associating myself with a particular group and others giving me the label (Shakespeare 2006: 71–4). At a particular time with a particular group, I could well be mainly supporting the goals of that group and proudly wear the badge, but this does not mean that this is all there is to me or that all my personal goals are compatible with the group's goals. Being labelled as a woman or as disabled, even if the person in question fits some of the stereotypical views concerning the group, will always only paint a partial picture of who that person is.

Given all the problems that community thinking leads to, I strongly agree with Tom Shakespeare (2006: 82) when he writes: 'The goal of disability politics should be to make impairment and disability irrelevant whenever possible, not to seek out and celebrate a separatist notion of disability pride based on an ethnic conception of disability identity.' This comment, if my analysis as presented in this chapter can be accepted, holds true of most politically motivated groups. Communities are 'good' to us both personally and on a political level, but there are serious limitations to their usefulness. In our responses to others, we should, as often as possible, see them as they are: as individual persons and not caricatures of the group we think they represent. And when fighting for the political agendas of oppressed groups, we should be mindful that there comes a time when setting 'us' against 'them' becomes self-defeating.

Acknowledgements

Earlier versions of this chapter were presented at the University of Reykjavik (Iceland) on 30 May 2007 and at the Annual International David Thomasma Bioethics Retreat in Cambridge on 18 June 2007. The author would like to thank the audiences on both occasions for inspirational comments and questions.

Notes

1 Please replace 'woman' with the category you have been associated with.
2 As many as 2 per cent of all children born alive could have ambiguous external genitalia in terms of their sex (Blackless *et al.* 2000: 151).

Bibliography

Amundson, R. (2005) 'Disability, Ideology and Quality of Life: A Bias in Biomedical Ethics', in D. Wasserman, J. Bickenback and R. Wachbroit (eds), *Quality of Life and Human Difference: Genetic Testing, Health Care, and Disability*, Cambridge: Cambridge University Press.

bat Tzeded, E. F. (2005) 'The Rights and Wrongs of Identity Politics and Sexual Identities', in M. B. Zinn, P. Hondagneu-Sotelo and M. A. Messner (eds), *Gender through the Prism of Difference*, 3rd edn, Oxford: Oxford University Press.

Blackless, M., Charuvastra, A., Derryk, A., Fausto-Sterling, A., Lausanne, K. and Lee, E. (2000) 'How Sexually Dimorphic Are We? Review and Synthesis', *American Journal of Human Biology*, 12: 151–66.

Gilligan, C. (1982) *In a Different Voice: Psychological Theory and Women's Development*, Cambridge, MA: Harvard University Press.

Glover, J. (1988) *I: The Philosophy and Psychology of Personal Identity*, London: Penguin.

Grillo, T. (2006), 'Anti-Essentialism and Intersectionality', in E. Hackett and S. Haslanger (eds), *Theorising Feminism: A Reader*, Oxford: Oxford University Press.

Hackett, E. and Haslanger, S. (eds) (2006) *Theorising Feminism: A Reader*, Oxford: Oxford University Press.

Longmore, P. K. (2003) *Why I Burned my Book and Other Essays on Disability*, Philadelphia, PA: Temple University Press.

Meyers, D. T. (2002) *Gender in the Mirror: Cultural Imagery and Women's Agency*, Oxford: Oxford University Press.

Parens, E. and Asch, A. (1999) 'The Disability Rights Critique of Prenatal Genetic Testing: Reflections and Recommendations', *Hastings Center Report*, 29: S1–S22.

Richards, J. R. (1982) *The Sceptical Feminist: A Philosophical Enquiry*, Harmondsworth: Penguin.

Shakespeare, T. (2006) *Disability Rights and Wrongs*, London and New York: Routledge.

Sparti, D. (2001) 'Making Up People: On Some Looping Effects of the Human Kind: Institutional Reflexivity or Social Control?', *European Journal of Social Theory*, 4: 331–49.

Swain, J. and French, S. (2000) 'Towards an Affirmation Model of Disability', *Disability and Society*, 15: 569–82.

Takala, T. and Häyry, M. (2004) 'Is Communitarian Thinking Altruistic?', *TRAMES*, 8: 276–86.

Young, I. M. (2006) 'Five Faces of Oppression', in E. Hackett and S. Haslanger (eds), *Theorising Feminism: A Reader*, Oxford: Oxford University Press.

Zinn, M. B. and Dill, B. T. (2005) 'Theorising Difference from Multiracial Feminism', in M. B. Zinn, P. Hondagneu-Sotelo and M. A. Messner (eds), *Gender through the Prism of Difference*, 3rd edn, New York and Oxford: Oxford University Press.

Part III
Ethics

Part II

Ethics

9 Cochlear implants, linguistic rights and 'open future' arguments

Patrick Kermit

Introduction

The technology of cochlear implants has led to considerable discussion in field of bioethics. There seems to be an unusually sharp division between those who support and those who oppose the new technology: proponents take the optimistic line that such implants will eliminate deafness in the future, while critics, some of whom are themselves deaf, reject the implant, claiming that Deaf[1] people are primarily members of a linguistic minority and not a group of disabled people in need of 'repair'. Some even accuse surgeons performing such implantations of attempting to commit ethnocide and of wanting to eradicate Deaf culture entirely.

Different participants in these discussions have developed distinct and opposing lines of argument. In this chapter, I examine and discuss a central argument of some notable supporters of the implant (Balkany *et al.* 1996; Davis 1997b; Levy 2002a, 2002b; Nunes 2001), arguing the view of the 'child's right to an open future'. This argument centres on the protection of autonomy, that is, on the 'child's right *not* to have her/his future options irrevocably foreclosed' (Takala 2003: 39). I will more closely examine this position presented by two leading participants in the current debate and ongoing discussions, Rui Nunes (2001) and Dena S. Davis (1997a). Both have argued that one of the consequences of failing to implant a deaf child is a curtailment of future options, and both establish the 'child's right to an open future' position as their main one. The above-mentioned Thomas Balkany *et al.* and Neil Levy utilise this argument as one among several others.

Joel Feinberg is the originator of the notion of a 'child's right to an open future'. The phrase is actually the title of his 1980 article where he first proposed the concept. Feinberg's argumentation is initially consistent, but when he then tries to account for the fact that children are in constantly changing phases as they struggle in moving towards adulthood, he fails to recognise that a child's development requires the fulfilment of certain other rights that fall outside his own schematic system. This is above all the 'right to language', something which carries with it essential implications for the 'right to social and cognitive development' in accordance with one's potential.

The result is a weakness in Feinberg's conceptualisation of 'an open future', a weakness that emerges more clearly and seriously when Nunes and Davis apply this concept to the controversy concerning paediatric cochlear implantation: there is a difference between becoming able to choose and the act of choosing itself. Feinberg's concern is with the first, that of protecting the child's future autonomy (Takala 2003). Nunes and Davis presuppose that the child with an implantation reaching adulthood is autonomous and able to choose his or her own way in life.

I contend that implantation and being facilitated with a cochlear implant can *in itself* pose a threat to the child's right to become autonomous, because this process of habilitation can be seen as violating the child's linguistic rights. Additionally, I will argue that the right to language is a basic human right, but will also claim that this right does not necessarily imply that a child cannot have more than one language.

The ethical debate on paediatric cochlear implantation

Different perspectives on deafness give rise to equally different opinions and perspectives in the ethical debate on paediatric cochlear implantation. From a physiological perspective, deafness is typically seen as a disadvantageous medical condition. Implanted persons still remain hard of hearing, but they may develop a capacity to understand speech through training and (re)habilitation. Prelingually deaf children who are implanted are expected not only to be able to perceive speech but also to develop spoken language. Thus, even though cochlear implants do not completely restore a deaf person's hearing, they are from a medical perspective considered a major advantage, if the individual's ability to perceive sounds is improved after such surgical intervention.

If one accepts the scientific discovery that signed languages are fully fledged natural languages (Stokoe 2005), capable of allowing exactly the same quality and range of communication as any spoken language, then one perhaps could and should also accept the position that Deaf people are members of a linguistic minority with a history and culture of their own. From this perspective, it would be wrong to consider deaf children as somehow in need of surgical intervention or habilitation; on the contrary, their most pressing need is the acquisition of a signed language. Because a signed language is primarily visual, the deaf child can acquire and learn to use it just as easily as a hearing child develops and uses a spoken language.

It should be clear by now why the cochlear implant has become a major ethical debate and discussion. From a medical viewpoint, deafness is defined first and foremost as an individual deficit, a pathological state of not being able to hear. This state of being can be explained with reference to aetiology: to undergo a profound or severe loss of hearing is normally brought about by illness, genetic deficiencies, or other health-related factors such as prenatal infection in the mother. Attempting to cure or ease the individual's condition by means of the latest technology would normally be thought of as ethically non-controversial, routine, perhaps even sought after and deemed praiseworthy.

On the other hand, if being Deaf means being a member of a linguistic minority with its own language and culture, then one can draw very different conclusions. To alter a child's cultural belongingness and identity by means of technology is ethically disturbing and problematic. If Deaf people are thought of as not being disabled but being instead part of a legitimate linguistic minority, it might be unethical to try to eradicate Deafness with cochlear implants. Some have even suggested that such implantations might hypothetically be compared to a treatment (actual or imaginary) whereby African Americans are offered the possibility of changing their skin colour from dark to light. This argument also suggests that the association between Deafness and disability relates to social (mis)perceptions rather than actual experience: in this case, the label of disability is a product of discrimination, and does not correspond to the daily realities of Deaf lives. The idea that Deaf people can be compared to something approaching an ethnic minority has been heavily disputed and rejected, among others by John Harris (2000).

'Open future' arguments and the question of deaf children's futures

Rui Nunes and Dena Davis both draw on Feinberg's argument of a 'right to an open future' when refuting Deaf claims that cochlear implantation poses a threat to prelingually deaf children. I would like to examine the different claims outlined so far by giving a brief presentation, beginning with the original understanding of 'an open future', and then more closely scrutinising the arguments of Nunes and Davis.

Feinberg's concept of the 'child's right to an open future'

Drawing on the work of the Enlightenment philosopher John Locke (1632–1704), Feinberg (1980) speaks of 'rights' as something one is born with. Locke, as with many other Enlightenment philosophers, sees man as a free and autonomous being. Thus, one's capacity for making free choices also makes one morally accountable for own actions and responsible to a great extent for what kind of person one becomes. It would follow that holding a child morally responsible for its own life and dispositions is obviously unreasonable. On the contrary, to bring up a child is to provide him or her with the means to gradually form an own identity and to increasingly assume adult responsibilities. Thus, even though all humans share the same rights because they all share the same humanity, as, for example, Immanuel Kant establishes (1983), rights are not equally ascribable to everyone. Some rights are shared by all human beings irrespective of age, such as the right to life and safety. Feinberg labels these as 'A-C-rights' (where A and C stand for 'Adult' and 'Child' respectively). Other rights, such as freedom of speech, and religious and political liberties, though they are shared by all humans, presuppose that the person exercising them is capable of making responsible and rational choices. Feinberg labels these rights 'A-rights'. Although no humans can be said not to share these A-rights, not all humans are capable of exercising them. Some individuals may be considered to be permanently incapacitated due to cognitive impairments. Children are also considered incapable of exercising these rights fully, but this is a temporary and partial incapacity: as a child matures, he or she will gradually assume more and more responsibility for one's own life and choices. Following along this line of thinking, Feinberg suggests identifying and recognising certain rights that are primarily ascribable to children, which he terms 'C-rights'. He divides these rights into two classes. First, there are 'dependency-rights' which he defines as ones relating to 'the child's dependence upon others for the basic instrumental goods of life – food, shelter, protection' (Feinberg 1980). And second, there are 'rights-in-trust' or 'anticipatory autonomy rights', which he relates to the child's rights to a future self-fulfilment and self-determination as an adult. To phrase it quite simply, he argues that 'rights-in-trust' can be summed up as the single 'right to an open future' (ibid.: 126).

This may leave one with the somewhat paradoxical impression that childhood is a relatively tranquil and undisturbed state of being, until that instant in time when the child becomes mature and takes on adult responsibilities and an adult identity. Feinberg recognises these paradoxes:

> If the grown-up offspring is to determine his own life, and be at least in large part the product of his own 'self-determination', he must already have a self fully formed and capable of doing the determining. But he cannot very well have determined *that* self on his own, because he would have to have been already a formed self to do that, and so on, *ad infinitum*.
>
> (ibid.: 147)

Feinberg points out that it is erroneous to think that we can identify a single moment in time when self-determination takes place. This carries with it the implication that it is impossible for parents to try to keep all future options for their child open at all times. More importantly, trying to do so would probably mean that the parents would have to neglect looking after some of the child's most important needs. This could for instance mean not raising a child with a certain set of values on the grounds that this would make it more difficult for the future adult to choose independently between different value systems. In order not to determine or otherwise limit the child's future ability to choose freely, one would have to try to raise the child in a state of total and unrestricted autonomy. But in his essay on 'the liberal dilemma', Hans Skjervheim argues that precisely such a scenario of unlimited freedom could easily result in the opposite: limitation and lack of freedom (1976). If freedom is conceived as the total absence of regulations or boundaries, a particular act or principle can never be regarded as more valuable or better than other alternative acts and principles. There is only one exception to this: the principle of unlimited freedom itself must be regarded as a valuable principle, but such a conception of freedom is only formal and offers no real guidance in life. If one tries to apply the formal principle to one's life, Skjervheim argues, the outcome could just as easily be nihilism and despair instead of meaning and happiness.

This constitutes a dilemma: no matter what decisions parents make on behalf of their children, their decisions affect what kind of open future the child will eventually have, by establishing the premises for what constitutes positive self-fulfilment for the child in the future:

> In a nutshell: the parents help create some of the interests whose fulfilment will constitute the child's own good. They cannot aim at an independent conception of the child's own good in deciding how to do this, because to some extent, the child's own good (self-fulfilment) depends on which interests the parents decide to create.
>
> (Feinberg 1980: 148)

Feinberg ends up by recommending a sort of cautious parental conduct. Recognising the fact that every parental incentive represents some sort of decision-making concerning future options, parents should carefully consider whose interests they have in mind when making decisions. If parents, for example, promote only their own ambitions and interests when considering suitable leisure activities ('Couldn't you play the piano instead of ice-hockey?'), this could mean closing down some of the child's future options, and additionally, doing so on the wrong premises.

Rui Nunes on cochlear implantation: securing the deaf child access to the hearing world

Nunes suggests what seems to be a moderate and reasonable compromise between those who are critical of and those who are favourable to paediatric cochlear implantation. He attempts to work out a balanced view on cochlear implants, but he rejects the notion that deaf children should be considered as members of the Deaf community and thus that they should learn a signed language:

> These children should be referred to as deaf (small letter). If it is true that a Deaf-World does exist, it is not clear that this cultural infusion is determined by the physiological handicap of deafness. It can be argued that the deaf child is not immediately, at birth, a member of the Deaf-World. It follows that there is no such thing as a birthright to be Deaf. It will be a member of that culture if, and only if, his or her parents take this option. Only then will this child be a Deaf child.
>
> (Nunes 2001: 343)

Nunes expresses sympathy and understanding for those who are concerned that the implant threatens the future of Deaf communities and Deaf culture. He also recognises the parental right to deny a deaf child implantation, particularly if the parents themselves are Deaf. Nevertheless, Nunes maintains that not to implant a

child may represent such a major barrier to future options that parents should not
be allowed to refuse implantation:

> If auditory (re)habilitation will in the future provide the necessary commu-
> nicative skills, in particular oral language acquisition, customs, values and
> attitudes of the hearing world should be regarded as necessary to accomplish
> a deaf child's right to an open future. ... It might follow that deaf children
> should not be deprived of cochlear implantation if it will be considered a
> technically safe and efficient process.
>
> (Nunes 2001)

In other words, Nunes is concerned that being Deaf primarily means to be cut off
from important aspects and areas of adult life. For example, it is statistically the case
that deaf people (there are few statistics available that deal with Deaf people only)
have lower levels of education and income than is the average for people with hearing (Harris *et al.* 1995; Nunes 2001).

Dena S. Davis on cochlear implantation: Deafness as an irrevocable limitation of future options

Even though Nunes allows some reservations for Deaf parents, he comes close to
implying that it is unjustifiable to refrain from implanting a child if such an intervention would give her or him sufficient communicative ability to enter the world
of speech. Dena S. Davis takes this argument one step further (1997a, 1997b). She
firmly states that the future is less open for a person who cannot hear: 'A hearing
person has a choice about whether to participate in DEAF culture, by learning
ASL [American Sign Language], attending social and cultural events, and so on.
A non-hearing person, however, is irrevocably cut off from large areas of the hearing
world' (Davis 1997a: 254).

She then goes on to argue that the choice left to the 'non-hearing person' to
become Deaf, is in itself limiting:

> [O]ne needs to think seriously about the limited opportunities that exist for
> even the most positively acculturated DEAF person. Marriage partners, con-
> versation partners, vocations, and avocations are severely limited. Yes, one
> can think of cultural minorities about whom the same could be said – e.g., the
> Amish or very Orthodox Jews – but these children can change their minds as
> adults and a significant percentage do so.
>
> (ibid.: 255)

Davis's conclusion is that refraining from implantation has a more negative and
constraining impact on the child's future options than other parental choices might
have, because the child will be confined to the Deaf world:

[E]very child has a 'right to an open future' ... in which she can choose her mate, her vocation, her religion, her reading material, her place of residence, and so forth. Because deafness severely limits the child's future *in an irrevocable fashion*, I cannot agree that parents act wrongly in 'curing' a child's deafness.

(ibid.: 255)

'Open future' arguments and the right to language

Nunes and Davis offer very convincing arguments, and it has to be said that the 'open future' position is at least intuitively very persuasive. But at this point I want to challenge Feinberg's concept, arguing that Feinberg leaves out important aspects of children's rights. Put in his own terminology, Feinberg overlooks the existence of a third class of 'C-rights' (previously described), the most important of which is the right to language. To put it very bluntly, I will claim that *the right to an open future* ceases to exist for a person who is not granted the full right to language.

Most people never have to concern themselves with the question of language as something one is entitled to have. In most majority communities, it is above all the single language they share that makes it possible for people to identify as a unity and a majority, and this is something one tends to take for granted. Likewise, most people don't have to reflect on the fact that they can usually speak their minds, freely, and without encumbrance.

This aspect of obviousness perhaps explains why linguistic rights are seldom codified, but it doesn't mean that they are never claimed. Many linguistic minorities today either struggle, or have a history of struggling, to gain recognition for their language (Eriksen 1991). In the fields of linguistics and philosophy, the question of linguistic rights has its own theoretical discourse (Chen 1998; Patten and Kymlicka 2003; Pennycook 1998; Skutnabb-Kangas 2002; Skutnabb-Kangas and Phillipson 1994). The United Nations (UN) Charter on Human Rights (1948) makes no reference to linguistic rights, but the United Nations Declaration on the Rights of Indigenous Peoples (2007: Article 13) does:

Indigenous peoples have the right to revitalise, use, develop and transmit to future generations their histories, languages, oral traditions, philosophies, writing systems and literatures, and to designate and retain their own names for communities, places and person.

The UN Convention on the Rights of the Child (1990) also claims such linguistic rights on behalf of children belonging to linguistic minorities. Deaf people have not tried to claim the rights of an indigenous nation, but nevertheless, their history has similarities with the history of numerous linguistic minorities worldwide. Reviewing patterns in the history of some of these minorities, the Norwegian anthropologist Thomas Hylland Eriksen points out how minorities often stand up to defend their languages when pressure from the outside world builds up:

> As the value of *air* becomes evident only from the moment the air becomes seriously polluted, so does the significance of belonging to 'a culture' – or a linguistic community – become an issue for reflection and political action only from the moment when the community seems threatened by imminent extinction. Such a development could provide a partial explanation for the linguistic revival witnessed in many parts of the world since the 1960s: Whereas minority languages such as Inuit, Saami and Breton were predicted to vanish within a generation in the early 1960s, subsequent developments have demonstrated a strong will to retain the languages, to revive them and to propagate their use in the modern bureaucratic sector of society.
>
> (Eriksen 1991: 42)

In order to understand this 'strong will to retain the languages', it is essential to recognise how one's language is tightly interwoven with one's identity and self-understanding. Members of majority communities are seldom forced to reflect on this aspect of their being in the same way that members of a minority often have to. When a language is threatened, it is not always something one can necessarily observe objectively from a distance. If it is *my* language which is under threat, my identity and my way of being in the world are also drawn into the line of fire. This is reflected in Eriksen's conclusion: 'those aspects of personal identity which are expressed through one's language, can be extremely important to the well-being of individuals. Linguistic rights should be seen as elementary human rights' (ibid. 42).

Although Eriksen's message is clearly relevant and helps us to understand why many Deaf people oppose cochlear implants, the point I want to make here is even more fundamental: there is a distinction between the right to have one particular language before another, and the fundamental right to language as a prerequisite for being in the world (see Chen 1998). In other words, the central issue here is not about the claims of a particular culture (Davis 1997a), but the right of the singular child to realise his or her lingual capacity (Corker 1998).

As previously mentioned, language is such a basic prerequisite for human activity that we do not usually reflect much on it. We owe much of the understanding of this inevitability of language to the Austrian philosopher Ludwig Wittgenstein, who famously expressed how the totality of our lives is defined by our lingual capacities in the sentence: '*Die Grenzen meiner Sprache* bedeuten die Grenzen meiner Welt' ('*The limits of my language* mean the limits of my world') (1992: 148). Wittgenstein's view was that my understanding of the world (and myself as a part of it) cannot normally[2] transcend my capacity to frame that world (and myself) through language. As we can never step outside the world or ourselves, we can never step outside of language. In expressing this, Wittgenstein tries to capture an essential truth about language: there is always something that eludes us when we try to frame the concept of language itself (1967). Hence, to try to say what language 'is' is a futile endeavour, since we can only capture parts of the concept. Despite knowing this, however, important aspects of language can still be identified.

Intuitively speaking, an obvious fact about language is that it enables us to communicate with each other.[3] Most people also agree that language allows us to extend the limits of our world through learning. But a third and less obvious aspect of language is how essential it is to the development and preservation of our selves: language is the medium which facilitates contact with the 'I' that constitutes us (Tugendhat 1979).

There are of course no sharp boundaries between these three aspects of what it means to have a language. Nevertheless, I want to draw attention to the fact that language is much more than just the ability to utter words in combination and to do so according to certain grammatical patterns. Language also involves much more than being able to speak one's mind to another person. Communicating through language is of course an immensely important element of its function, but it is far from being the only one. We do not have language only in order to communicate with others. Language is something that enables me *to articulate my self to myself.* This understanding of my specific way of being in the world is accessible not only to others, but first of all to me, through my lingual representation of myself. In other words, language is a prerequisite for any formation of an identity, for self-understanding and for autonomy.

This is also recognised in fields of science other than philosophy: linguistics, educational sciences and psychology have become ever more aware of the intimate connection between language and cognitive development (Lahey 1988). No sharp division can be made between these two forms of development, since each presupposes the existence of the other (Mead 1912; Mead 1913; Vygotsky 1978). Research in these fields has also revealed another interesting thing about language acquisition: the importance of children's peer interaction (Frønes 1998; Matre 1997). There are many indications that a child's primary source of language is obtained through interaction with age-peers and not through interaction with the adults around her or him who 'know' the language. This might not be unreasonable if one rejects the oversimplified view that language is about knowing words and how to combine them grammatically. Knowing a language is first of all about knowing how to use it (Wittgenstein 1967) as a tool for actions (both cognitive and communicative). When children interact, it is unclear when 'learning to speak' starts and 'learning to act' (or 'learning to learn' for that matter) stops. These are all aspects of the same developing process.

From this perspective, it is impossible to impede the child's right to language without also denying a range of other rights one usually recognises. The conclusion, then, is that it is only if you develop your full linguistic potential as a child that your future can be fully open.

It is somewhat odd that Feinberg overlooks the importance of language when he discusses children's rights. Even in 1980 when he wrote his article, the philosophy of language was a well-established branch of philosophy. On the other hand, as previously mentioned, language is such an implicit entity in our lives that it is often taken for granted. The sciences are no exception, something pointed out by the German philosopher Johann Gottlieb Fichte as early as the late eighteenth century: '[Fichte] delighted in calling attention to the unavoidable circularity of all systematic explanations and to the need for even the most "pre-suppositionless" science to begin by presupposing such things as natural language and the ordinary rules of reflection' (Breazeale 1991: 528).

Feinberg is vulnerable to this kind of criticism. His previously discussed attempt to avoid the circle whereby adult self-determination always presupposes an autonomous self is doomed to be unsuccessful as long as the acquisition of a primary language is a prerequisite for ever becoming capable of self-determination. The whole concept of a 'right to an open future' can be said to suffer from the lack of a more thorough evaluation of a child's basic need for language. The right to develop language and one's cognitive and social capacities cannot be characterised either as a dependent 'C-right' or a 'right-in-trust'. It seems instead that Feinberg underestimates the importance of language acquisition as a process that should not go wrong:

> The standard sort of loving upbringing and a human social environment in the earliest years will be like water added to dehydrated food, filling it out and actualising its stored-in tendencies. Then the child's earliest models for imitation will make an ineluctable mark on him. He will learn one language rather than another, for instance, and learn it with a particular accent and inflection. His own adult linguistic style will be in the making virtually from the beginning.
>
> (Feinberg 1980: 149)

Feinberg expresses a natural confidence in the possible congenital ability of the child to acquire language. In most cases, I believe he is correct: even though language acquisition is not an uncomplicated project, it usually ends well for most children – but, the result is by no means automatic, and not all children manage the process successfully. There is nothing to be taken for granted when it comes to language development, and the 'standard sort of loving upbringing and a human social environment' do not necessarily guarantee success; at best, they only provide some necessary prerequisites. Previous research on children with cochlear implants, together with the historical knowledge we have about the experiences of deaf and hard-of-hearing children, suggests that some of these children never get to realise their full lingual potential in spite of a loving family and perfectly adequate social support.

The life experiences of deaf and hard-of-hearing people

Before cochlear implantation became an established and available medical procedure in the industrialised parts of the world, children with hearing impairments would normally have been labelled 'deaf' or 'hard-of-hearing', depending on their medically determined hearing status. Since the end of the nineteenth century, an overarching goal in the education of children with hearing impairments in most western countries has been the production and perception of speech. As the varying degrees of hearing loss made this a challenging task, both deaf and hard-of-hearing children were normally identified as requiring some kind of 'special needs education': deaf children (who obviously had the greatest difficulties in perceiving sounds) would mostly attend deaf schools, while children who were hard-of-hearing would either attend special schools for the hard-of-hearing or mainstream schools where there was some level of support (for example, in the form of technical aids).

It was not until the second half of the twentieth century that the slow process of recognising signed languages as fully fledged languages began to emerge. Deaf children would nevertheless sign mostly to each other and with signing adults at the deaf schools. Even in those deaf schools where signed language was not acknowledged as a suitable tool for educational purposes, the schools still functioned as important places for the passing on of signing to new generations of deaf children, thus providing a central platform for Deaf culture. The educational results attained by those who attended deaf schools were still poor, especially since many of the students had to rely on lip-reading in order to decipher what the teacher was saying.

From a 'special needs education perspective', the hard-of-hearing students were normally believed and expected to be more successful than the deaf students. With adult support and training, the hard-of-hearing children could pick up speech with different degrees of success, with the challenges they faced depending very much on their hearing. For these children a signed language was considered superfluous and unnecessary, since the assumption was that sign languages were inferior to spoken ones. For those who did not start to produce speech, there was always the possibility of being transferred to the deaf school, whereas the deaf students who picked up speech and showed good progress would often be transferred in the other direction (Kermit 2006).

Still, from an educational perspective the students who could speak would be considered the more successful ones, and those with the best prospects for the future. When Deaf and hard-of-hearing people themselves tell about their school experiences, another story often emerges. Even though Deaf people tell about lost opportunities that were a result of the poor outcome of their education, they still tell about friends and of a rich social life at school. Hard-of-hearing people who attended mainstream schools often tell an opposite story, that of having managed to cope in the classroom, but at the same time suffering from loneliness, not having friends and being assigned an inferior role in social settings with peers (Brunnberg 2003; Grønlie 2005; Kruth 1996; Ladd 2003; Padden and Humphries 1988).

The mechanisms which cause problems for the interaction of hard-of-hearing children with their hearing peers are complex, but part of the difficulty has to do with the question of what it means to acquire and 'know' a language. Even if an adult understands the spoken language of a hard-of-hearing child and even if the child shows pragmatic skills and dialogue competence when interacting with the adult, these abilities need not be transferable to the sphere of the child's

interactions with hearing peers. As previously mentioned, children do not interact together in the same manner as an adult and a child (Frønes 1998), and it is
possible that the hard-of-hearing child struggles to obtain vital experiences in
peer interaction, something that constantly disables her or him in efforts to talk
with peers. An adult who interacts with a hard-of-hearing child can be supportive,
co-operative and reflect on limitations in the child's hearing. Hearing peers don't
necessarily have these cooperative skills and may be incapable of modifying their
communication in ways to make it easier for the hard-of-hearing child to understand (Kermit *et al.* 2005; Wray *et al.* 1997). The implication then is that even
if many hard-of-hearing children seem perfectly capable of speaking and also
understanding most of the things said by others, some of these children may be
cut of from the possibility of acquiring language in the more fundamental ways
described above, ways crucially related to self-image, identity and cognition.

This might well be the case for many cochlear-implanted children as well. Even
though these children can only with certain reservations be compared with hard-
of-hearing children, there are many studies that very strongly suggest that some
implanted children experience problems interacting through language (Mukari
et al. 2007; Tye-Murray 2003; Wie 2005). The exact numbers are somewhat
unclear, since most outcome studies of cochlear implantation focus only on
speech perception and speech production (Thoutenhoofd *et al.* 2005), something
which, at least in this context, is a very narrow definition of language. Still, if
some implanted children run the risk of not acquiring a language, this is a matter
of considerable ethical importance.

The bilingual approach and the possibility of having more than one language

If it is not possible to be certain that a high percentage of implanted children can
have their right to language fulfilled by learning to speak and perceive speech by
hearing it, it might be reasonable to claim that teaching implanted children a signed
language is the only ethically defendable way to secure their linguistic rights: the
implanted child would have easier access to a signed language. At least in theory,
a signed language is something a child can learn and produce with no more effort
than most other hearing children learn a spoken language. The child's need for
symmetric peer interaction would also be more easily achievable among other
signing children, as the school experiences of Deaf people previously referred to
seem to indicate.

On the other hand, both Nunes and Davis are clearly correct in pointing out
that options are limited if one has no access to the language of the majority community. This begs the question: is the attempt to have both a signed and a spoken
language a reasonable and ethically defensible one?

Research on bilingual children with two spoken languages is extensive and
generally indicates that children have a more than sufficient ability to master several languages, something which at the same time can be potentially rewarding
for cognitive development. The degree of proficiency in the two languages may,

however, vary depending on different factors: some are so proficient that it is difficult to identify which of the two languages is primary. At the opposite end of the scale, a child can have high levels of proficiency in a primary language and a capacity for using another language in certain contexts (Engen and Kulbrandstad 2004). It is not necessarily correct to characterise children with high proficiency in two languages as being somehow 'more bilingual' or 'successful' than other bilingual children. Contextual factors (such as where one lives, educational settings, and upbringing in a mono or bilingual family) influence what kind of demand or expectations exist for high proficiency in more than one language.[4]

It is also possible for a child to have a bilingual capacity where the two different languages together satisfy what another child gets from speaking only one language. This latter category, termed 'functional bilingualism' in Norway (Engen and Kulbrandstad 2004, my translation), is especially relevant and interesting for the situation of hearing-impaired children. Theoretically speaking, an implanted child with such a bilingual ability could have 'the best of both worlds': on the one hand, sharing vital lingual experiences through interacting with signing peers (experiences which are more difficult to have with speaking peers), and on the other hand, if the child can understand a speaking teacher, instructor or trainer, this opens up a range of additional possibilities. In educational settings, being able to speak is a valuable asset for developing reading and writing skills. And this approach has a further advantage: it does not prescribe the same cure for everybody, but can be adjusted to suit the individual child, thus letting her or him show the way: some implanted children may choose to shift the weight in the direction of signing, others in the direction of speech. (And this can in fact happen independently of clinical hearing status, for there are Deaf people who have better hearing than others who think of themselves as hard-of-hearing.) Even if he doesn't comment directly on the crucial importance of language, preparing children to make their own choices is actually very much in line with what Feinberg suggests parents should do.

Concluding remarks

My main objective in this chapter has been to uncover weaknesses in the arguments of Rui Nunes and Dena Davis, and thus hopefully contribute to the ethical discourse on paediatric cochlear implantation. As both Nunes and Davis rely very heavily on Feinberg's concept of a 'right to an open future', it has been necessary to analyse this concept as well. I have done so in order to unveil and pinpoint where problems arise when Feinberg's thoughts are applied to the debate on cochlear implants.

By not paying particular attention to the child's right to language and to the associated cognitive development as a self-contained class of 'C-rights', Feinberg obscures his own main objective – namely, to show the difference between being and becoming autonomous, between choosing freely and becoming able to choose. This causes an unfortunate lack of clarity as to how the concept of the 'child's right to an open future' should be interpreted. Both Nunes and Davis exploit the concept's rhetorical strength (who would deny a child an open future?), and because the concept is so vague, they can do so without having to discuss – as I have done here – what the best possible development for a deaf child might really be.

In her argumentation, Davis seems to be unaware that deaf children do not by any means become hearing the minute they are implanted. One almost suspects that Davis argued under the tacit assumption that future implants would cure deafness instantly without the need for habilitation (as some other theorists have done, e.g., Levy 2002b). Nunes shows greater awareness that the implant is not an instant cure, but he also demonstrates a very instrumental approach to the question of language. His only demand is that 'it must be scientifically proved that the implanted child not only has audiological perception but also acquires communicative ability' (Nunes 2001: 345).

As I have argued, it is not obvious that 'communicative ability' is equivalent to everything associated with 'having a language'. On the contrary, the notion of a language as only a means of communication again ignores the fact that languages are bound up in very significant ways with self-image, identity and cognition. Nunes' demand does not satisfy these latter aspects of what it means to have language. A person may have communicative abilities but still not develop all of the attributes linked to self-articulation.

Even though Nunes makes some allowances for Deaf parents, he comes close to implying that it is unjustifiable not to implant a child if the implant gives her or him this 'communicative ability'. Davis is even more explicit, implying that it is ethically questionable not to implant because, in her view, the future is more open for a person who can choose between being a member of a Deaf or a hearing community than it is for a deaf person who cannot choose.

When it comes to the discussion of lingual rights and bilingual possibilities, the positions that I have reviewed in this chapter could in fact be totally reversed: if there is even a small chance that habilitation after implantation by means of only one spoken language could irrevocably violate children's right to language and their subsequent cognitive and social development, we should most likely refrain from such monolingual habilitation on the grounds that it is unethical. If it is the case that deaf implanted children need to make an extra effort in order to learn to perceive speech, then this can only be defended ethically if the time and effort required do not prevent the child from acquiring a signed language as well. For the bilingual deaf child, the cochlear implant may very well be a useful device that makes it easier to perceive speech.

This way of arguing offers a consistent approach to the question of how the deaf child's right to an open future can be better ensured. As a technical device, the implant in itself poses no threat to the child's future autonomy, but if the child's habilitation with the implant violates her/his right to language, the child's future may in the worst case be irrevocably closed in both the hearing and the Deaf worlds. Hence, the implant should only be used in ways that do not threaten the child's language acquisition. A bilingual approach seems to be the most advantageous, allowing the child to have 'the best of both worlds'. Seen in this context, the implant may very well be a useful asset to the child, albeit no more than a technical aid that helps with those parts of spoken language that require speech perception and speech production.

It is when the notion of a right to language meets the empirical understanding that cochlear implants may threaten a child's ability to acquire language in the full sense, that the ethical aspects of cochlear implantation and the weakness of the open future argument become clear. The way that Nunes and Davis conceive of both the concept of language and the concept of an 'open future' is narrow and over-simplified. The concept of an 'open future' is not about having the maximum amount of choices as an adult: it is about becoming a free, rational and autonomous agent. The latter is only possible for the child who is allowed to develop and realise her/his potential to the full – a process that presupposes language as a basic prerequisite.

Notes

1 I follow the custom of differentiating between the medical condition of being *deaf* (which is written with a lower case 'd') and being a member of a signing community (where *Deaf* is written with a capital 'D') (Padden and Humphries 1988).
2 Wittgenstein probably does not fully exclude the possibility that I can recognise truths beyond the grasp of language, but this discussion falls outside this text.
3 Something else that Wittgenstein demonstrates, and which is less intuitive, is that it is impossible to have a private language you do not share with anyone else (1967).
4 For example, most Norwegian children have some proficiency in English because English is taught at school, and in a 'weak' sense they may thus be characterised as bilingual. Many of these children can use this ability in activities such as global interactive games on the Internet and will not feel any need for a higher level of proficiency. A child growing up with a Norwegian mother and a father who is a native speaker of English may quite naturally develop bilingually with high proficiency in two languages.

Bibliography

Balkany, T., Hodges, A. V. and Goodman, K. W. (1996) 'Ethics of Cochlear Implantation in Young Children', *Otolaryngology, Head and Neck Surgery*, 114: 748–55.

Breazeale, D. (1991) 'Why Fichte now?', *Journal of Philosophy*, 88: 524–31.

Brunnberg, E. (2003) *Vi bytte våra hörande skolekamrater mot döva: förändring av hörselskadade barns identitet och självförtroende vid byte av språklig skolmilö [We Exchanged Our Hearing School-Friends with Deaf Ones: Changes in the Identity and Self-Confidence for Hearing-Impaired Children by Changing the Language of School-Environments]*, Örebro, Sweden: Örebro University.

Chen, A. H. Y. (1998) 'The Philosophy of Language Rights', *Language Sciences*, 20: 45–54.

Corker, M. (1998) *Deaf and Disabled, or Deafness Disabled? Towards a Human Rights Perspective*, Buckingham: Open University Press.

Davis, D. S. (1997a) 'Cochlear Implants and the Claims of Culture? A Response to Lane and Grodin', *Kennedy Institute of Ethics Journal*, 7: 253–8.

—— (1997b) 'Genetic Dilemmas and the Child's Right to an Open Future', *Hastings Centre Report*, 27: 7–15.

Engen, T. O. and Kulbrandstad, L. A. (2004) *Tospråklighet, minoritetsspråk og minoritetsundervisning [Bilingualism, Minority Language, and Education of Minorities]*, Oslo: Gyldedal Akademisk.

Eriksen, T. H. (1991) *Languages at the Margins of Modernity: Linguistic Minorities and the Nation-State*, Oslo: International Peace Research Institute (PRIO).

Feinberg, J. (1980) 'The Child's Right to an Open Future', in W. Aiken and H. LaFollette (eds), *Whose Child? Children's Rights, Parental Authority, and State Power*, Totowa, NJ: Littlefield, Adams and Co.

Frønes, I. (1998) *De likeverdige: om sosialisering og de jevnaldrendes betydning [The Equals: Socialisation and the Significance of Peer-relationships]*, Oslo: Universitets-forlaget.

Grønlie, S. M. (2005) *Uten hørsel? En bok om hørselshemming [Without Hearing? A Book about Hearing Impairment]*, Bergen: Fagbokforlaget.

Harris, J. (2000) 'Is There a Coherent Social Conception of Disability?' *Journal of Medical Ethics*, 26: 95–100.

Harris, J. P., Anderson, J. P., and Novak, R. (1995) 'An Outcome Study of Cochlear Implants in Deaf Patients: Audiologic, Economic, and Quality-of-Life Changes', *Archives of Oto-laryngology Head and Neck Surgery*, 121: 398–404.

Kant, I. (1983) 'Grunnlegging av moralens metafysikk (Grundlegung zur Metaphysik der Sitten) [Fundamental Principles of the Metaphysics of Morals]', in E. Storheim (ed.), *Moral, politikk og historie*, Oslo: Universitetsforlaget.

Kermit, P. (2006) 'Tegnspråk og anerkjennelsen av døve som en språklig minoritet [Sign Language and the Recognition of Deaf People as a Linguistic Minority]', in S. R. Jørgensen and R. L. Anjum (eds), *Tegn som språk: en antologi om tegnspråk [Signs as Language: An Anthology about Sign Language]*, Oslo: Gyldendal Akademisk.

Kermit, P., Holm, A., and Mjøen, O. M. (2005) *Cochleraimplantat i et tospråklig og etisk perspektiv [Cochlear Implantation in a Bilingual and Ethnic Perspective]* (Report No. 14), Trondheim, Norway: University-College of Sør-Trøndelag, Department of Teaching and Interpreter Education.

Kruth, L. (1996) *En tyst värld – full av liv [A Silent World: Full of Life]*, Örebro: SIH Läromedel.

Ladd, P. (2003) *Understanding Deaf Culture: In Search of Deafhood*, London: Cromwell Press.

Lahey, M. (1988) *Language Disorders and Language Development*, Basingstoke: Macmillan.

Levy, N. (2002a) 'Deafness, Culture and Choice', *Journal of Medical Ethics*, 28: 284–5.

—— (2002b) 'Reconsidering Cochlear Implants: The Lessons of Martha's Vineyard', *Bioethics*, 16: 134–53.

Matre, S. (1997) 'Munnlege tekstar hos barn: ein studie av barn 5–8 år i dialogisk samspell [Oral Texts among Children: A Study of Children Aged 5–8 in Dialogic Interaction]', unpublished doctoral dissertation, Trondheim: Norwegian University of Science and Technology.

Mead, G. H. (1912) 'The Mechanism of Social Consciousness', *Journal of Philosophy, Psychology and Scientific Methods*, 9: 401–6.

—— (1913) 'The Social Self', *Journal of Philosophy, Psychology and Scientific Methods*, 10: 374–80.

Mukari, S. Z., Ling, L. N., and Ghani, H. A. (2007) 'Educational Performance of Pediatric Cochlear Implant Recipients in Mainstream Classes', *International Journal of Pediatric Otorhinolaryngology*, 71: 231–40.

Nunes, R. (2001) 'Ethical Dimension of Paediatric Cochlear Implantation', *Theoretical Medicine and Bioethics*, 22: 337–49.

Padden, C. and Humphries, T. (1988) *Deaf in America: Voices from a Culture*, Cambridge, MA: Harvard University Press.

Patten, A. and Kymlicka, W. (2003) 'Introduction: Language Rights and Political Theory: Context, Issues, and Approaches', in W. Kymlicka and A. Patten (eds), *Language Rights and Political Theory*, Oxford: Oxford University Press.

Pennycook, A. (1998) 'The Right to Language: Towards a Situated Ethics of Language Possibilities', *Language Sciences*, 20: 73–87.

Skjervheim, H. (1976) *Deltakar og tilskodar og andre essays [Participant and Audience and Other Essays]*, Oslo: Tanum-Norli.

Skutnabb-Kangas, T. (2002) 'Marvelous Human Rights Rhetoric and Grim Realities: Language Rights in Education', *Journal of Language, Identity and Education*, 1: 179–205.

Skutnabb-Kangas, T. and Phillipson, R. (1994) 'Linguistic Human Rights, Past and Present', in R. Phillipson and T. Skutnabb-Kangas (eds), *Linguistic Human Rights: Overcoming Linguistic Discrimination*, Berlin and New York: Mouton de Gruyter.

Stokoe, W. C., Jr. (2005) 'Sign Language Structure: An Outline of the Visual Communication Systems of the American Deaf', *Journal of Deaf Studies and Deaf Education*, 10: 3–37.

Takala, T. (2003) 'The Child's Right to an Open Future and Modern Genetics', in B. Almond and M. Parker (eds), *Ethical Issues in the New Genetics: Are Genes Us?*, Aldershot: Ashgate.

Thoutenhoofd, E. D., Archbold, S. M., Gregory, S., Lutman, M. E., Nikolopoulos, T. P. and Sach, T. H. (2005) *Paediatric Cochlear Implantation*, London: Whurr Publishers.

Tugendhat, E. (1979) *Selbstbewußtsein und Selbstbestimmung: Sprachanalytische Interpretationen [Self-Consciousness and Self-Determination: A Linguistic Interpretation]*, Frankfurt: Suhrkamp Verlag.

Tye-Murray, N. (2003) 'Conversational Fluency of Children who Use Cochlear Implants', *Ear and Hearing*, 24: 82S–9S.

United Nations (1948) *Universal Declaration of Human Rights*, New York: United Nations. Available at < http://www.un.org/Overview/rights.html > (accessed 5 February 2008).

—— (1990) *Convention on the Rights of the Child*, New York: United Nations. Available at < http://www.unhchr.ch/html/menu3/b/k2crc.htm > (accessed 5 February 2008).

—— (2007) *United Nations Declaration on the Rights of Indigenous Peoples*, New York: United Nations. Available at < http://daccessdds.un.org/doc/UNDOC/GEN/N06/512/07/PDF/N0651207.pdf?OpenElement > (accessed 5 February 2008).

Vygotsky, L. (1978) *Mind in Society: The Development of Higher Psychological Processes*, Cambridge, MA: Harvard University Press.

Wie, O. B. (2005) *Kan Døve Bli Hørende? En Kartlegging av de Hundre Første Barna med Cochleaimplantat i Norge*, [Can the Deaf Become Hearing? A Survey of the First Hundred Children with Cochlear Implants in Norway], Oslo: Unipub forlag.

Wittgenstein, L. (1967) *Philosophical Investigations*, Oxford: Blackwell.

—— (1992) *Tractatus Logico-Philosophicus*, London and New York: Routledge.

Wray, D., Flexer, C., and Vaccaro, V. (1997) 'Classroom Performance of Children who Are Deaf or Hard of Hearing and Who Learned Spoken Communication through the Auditory-Verbal Approach: An Evaluation of Treatment Efficacy', *Volta Review*, 99: 107.

10 The moral contestedness of selecting 'deaf embryos'

Matti Häyry

Introduction

My aim in this chapter is to study the ethics of selecting 'deaf embryos' and to argue that the deep moral disagreement visible in the contemporary bioethical debate about the possibility should be recognised and accepted, not drowned in feuds. To begin, I will describe, in the first two sections, the background to the practice in emerging reproductive technologies and sketch the main moral and legal stands that can be taken in its assessment and regulation. I will then go on to examine, in the third and fourth sections, the moral justifications that have been given for the two competing views on the issue: the Medical View and the Social View. The first of these states that selecting 'deaf embryos' is morally dubious although it should, as far as the law is concerned, be left to the discretion of the parents. The second contends that the practice is morally unproblematic or even commendable but agrees that the law should not interfere with parental choice. Following the ethical analyses, the permissive legal stance, potentially shared by the two views, is outlined in the fifth section, and stock is taken of the argumentation so far in the sixth. Problems identified in the moral cases for the Medical and Social Views are considered in the seventh and eighth sections. My conclusion in the final two sections is that to avoid directive pressure on potential parents, both parties should admit that the choice to select 'deaf embryos' is not obviously right or wrong, but genuinely morally contested.

The techniques and their uses

The reproductive and diagnostic techniques needed to select 'deaf embryos' are in vitro fertilisation (IVF), pre-implantation genetic diagnosis (PGD), embryo selection (ES), and embryo transfer (ET).

In IVF, separately retrieved eggs and sperm are incubated together in a petri dish until, in successful cases, fertilisation occurs. In PGD, one cell of the six-to-eight-cell embryo is usually removed on day three after fertilisation, and genetic analyses are performed by one or more methods. The preferred embryos are then selected and transferred into the uterus of the potential mother for implantation. IVF has been used since 1978 and currently over 1 per cent of all pregnancies in the United Kingdom and the United States are conceived this way; in Denmark, this figure is over 4 per cent. The first PGD births occurred in 1990 and although the exact numbers are not known, the practice seems to be gaining in popularity.

IVF and ET are primarily used in clinical settings as an infertility treatment for people who cannot have children by other means. PGD and ES can also be employed in this context: the chances of a successful pregnancy can be improved by screening embryos to be transferred for their survival and implantation qualities. Additionally, PGD and ES have been developed to rule out genetic conditions in unborn individuals. If genetic mutations can be detected in time, terminations and selection can be used to eliminate monogenic diseases (conditions believed to be caused by a single gene) and the probability of polygenic diseases (conditions caused by a combination of hereditary and environmental factors). This has been seen as an opportunity to increase parental choice and, where PGD is used, as a way to reduce abortions. The ultimate aims include the prevention of harm and suffering and the production of healthier members of society.

The focus of this chapter is on a different practice, though – the attempt to use these techniques in order to create deaf offspring (cf. Robertson 2003). In a famous case in 2001, a deaf lesbian couple wanted to have deaf babies, arguing that their condition is not a medical affliction but a culture that they want to share with their children. Their way of pursuing this was to use a sperm donor with five generations of deafness in his family (Spriggs 2002). With appropriate advances in science, the chosen methods could conceivably have been PGD and ES. Although the possibility of success is currently unclear, a review conducted in the United States in 2006 revealed that 3 per cent of the PGDs provided by 137 IVF clinics were to 'select for a disability' (Baruch *et al.* 2007).

The case, the options and the stands

The hypothetical case to be considered in my analysis is the following. Six embryos have been produced by IVF, and PGD reveals that three of them are 'deaf' and three are 'hearing'. Three of the embryos can be implanted, and the question facing the decision makers is, which ones? One option would be to select all the 'deaf' embryos. Another would be to select all the 'hearing' embryos. Yet another option would be to 'let nature take its course', either by ignoring the information or by deliberately implanting a mixture of 'deaf' and 'hearing' embryos. (The attributes 'deaf' and 'hearing' are placed in scare quotes here and throughout the chapter as predicates of embryos, because embryos do not have the proper organs and capacities for hearing in any case. The expression refers to an increased probability of the ensuing individual being deaf or hearing.)

The rightness and wrongness of decisions like this can be assessed both morally and legally. It can be said that a decision to choose a specified course of action is:

- *morally wrong*, in which case the moral reasons for making it are outweighed by the moral reasons against making it; or
- *morally contested*, in which case the moral reasons for and against it have approximately equal weight; or
- *morally right*, in which case the moral reasons against making it are outweighed by the moral reasons for making it.

In a similar vein, it can be argued that a specified course of action should be:

- *legally prohibited*; or
- *legally permitted*; or
- *legally required.*

The relationship between moral and legal judgments can be seen in many ways. To sketch the main approaches to the matter: natural law theorists believe that the law should reflect morality at least to the degree that serious moral wrongs are legally prohibited regardless of their consequences; legal positivists think that law should be kept completely separate from moral considerations; and liberals normally hold that morality should not be enforced by law unless immoral actions can be expected to inflict harm on innocent bystanders.. The view taken here is, more concretely, that legal prohibitions and requirements can justifiably be backed up with state-enforced financial or physical sanctions (fines, imprisonment, and the like), while moral condemnations and obligations cannot.

Two main stands have been taken in the recent literature regarding the morality and legality of selecting 'deaf embryos'. These are presented schematically in Table 10.1.

The Medical View proceeds from the dual idea that deafness is a disability and that disabilities are conditions that individuals have and are harmed by. The Social View, in contrast, starts from the assumption that disabilities are human-made constructs predicated to individuals and groups on the basis of cultural perceptions (e.g. Vehmas and Mäkelä 2008). The moral bases of these notions will be examined in the next three sections.

The moral case for the Medical View

One of the first principles of traditional medical ethics is to 'do no harm' (Gillon 1985: 80–85). Medical interventions should benefit individual patients by removing or relieving ailments or by preventing them from occurring or getting worse. If an intervention is also expected to harm a patient, the harm should be outweighed by the anticipated benefit. For instance, although the loss of a limb is generally seen as a harm, an amputation can in certain cases be justified, if it probably will save the life of the patient.

The application of this principle to reproductive choices has always been controversial. Abortions have been defended on the grounds that they would prevent harm to pregnant women, but the comparison of harm inflicted on two different individuals falls outside the original, more individual-oriented, scope of the 'do no harm' rule. If the potential child is taken into account, and if life is seen as a benefit, another kind of balancing exercise seems to be needed.

The tool for weighing harms and benefits across individuals can be found in consequentialist ethics. According to this type of thinking, an action is morally right when it is aimed at producing more net good than any other alternative action open to the decision maker at the time of the choice (Häyry 1994, 2007). The model has been extended to reproductive choices by two stipulations. The

Table 10.1 The Medical View and the Social View

↓ / →	Selecting the 'deaf embryos' is / should be		
	legally prohibited	**legally permitted**	**legally required**
morally wrong	Medical View		
morally contested			
morally right		Social View	

first states that individuals, especially unborn ones, are 'replaceable'. It does not intrinsically matter which one of two possible human beings will actually come into existence: a potential life can be replaced by another potential life without violating any rights or absolute moral rules (Hare 1976). The second asserts that when a choice between future people is made, we should exercise 'procreative beneficence' and seek to create the best individuals we can. The idea is that, with the number of persons remaining the same, better human beings would make up a better world than worse human beings (Savulescu 2001; cf. Häyry 2004a; Parker 2007). (The distinction between 'better' and 'worse' human beings will be questioned in due course.)

The most vocal defence of the Medical View in the context of selecting 'deaf embryos' has come from John Harris, and it combines features of the traditional medical ethos and the more specifically consequentialist approach (Harris 2000, 2001, 2007: 102–103; cf. Häyry 1999; Takala 2003). The mixture is not entirely unproblematic, since the 'do no harm' rule is compatible with a variety of other principles, including the non-outcome-oriented versions of the principles of autonomy, justice, and dignity, while consequentialism sees outcomes as the only criterion of rightness and wrongness. It is therefore best to examine the two strands of justification separately.

Harris presents his 'medical ethics' argument in the form of four scenarios which he sees as morally similar. These are:

• deafening a hearing child;
• not curing an illness that would make a hearing child deaf;
• not making a deaf newborn hearing when there is a chance to do so;
• selecting a 'deaf embryo'.

Two claims need to be made, and have been made by Harris, to turn this list into an argument. The first is that deafening a hearing child is always clearly wrong, and something that a doctor should never do. The second is that the items on the list resemble each other so closely as to be equivalent or at least almost equivalent in moral terms. Since deafening a hearing child would be wrong and since selecting a 'deaf embryo' is morally on a par with it, it is also wrong (Harris 2000: 97, 2007: 102–103). Both choices would violate the 'do no harm' rule.

The consequentialist case for the Medical View is based on the assumptions that deafness is a disability and disabilities are harms. Disability, according to

Harris (2001: 384), is 'a condition that someone has a strong rational preference not to be in and one that is in some sense a harmed condition'. As a test, Harris suggests that 'a harmed condition is one which if a patient was brought unconscious into the accident or emergency department of a hospital in such a condition and it could be reversed or removed the medical staff would be negligent if they failed to reverse or remove it'. As examples he gives deafness and the 'loss of the bottom joint of the little finger'. When it comes to choosing among the six embryos, he argues that the potential mother 'has a reason to do what she can to ensure that the individual she chooses is as good an individual as she can make it' and 'therefore [she has a reason] to choose the embryo that is not already harmed in any particular way [...]' (ibid.: 385).[1] To prevent future disability and harm, and thereby to produce the best possible individual, the potential mother has a moral duty *not* to choose the 'deaf embryos'.

Both lines of argument for the Medical View will be critically reconsidered in the seventh section of this chapter.

The moral case for the Social View

The moral justification of the Social View needs two elements. The first is to challenge the idea that deafness in particular and conditions associated with disabilities in general can be counted as harms. The second is to build a positive case for selecting 'deaf' as opposed to 'hearing' embryos. Success on both fronts would imply that the moral reasons for selecting 'deaf embryos' can outweigh the moral reasons against it, which is the criterion of rightness assumed above (in the second section). An additional aspect, often emphasised by disability scholars, is an explanation of the disadvantages of 'being different' in terms of social reactions and constructs rather than medically definable impairments.

Defenders of the Social View have countered the 'harmed condition' argument by drawing attention to the experiences people actually have, as opposed to the 'rational preferences' they ought to have (according to consequentialist thinkers such as Harris). The lesbian women who wanted to have deaf babies, Sharon Duchesneau and Candace McCullough, for instance, stated in the media that deafness for them is an identity, culture, and community, not a medical problem or a harmful condition (Mundy 2002). Others in the deaf community have argued to the same effect that 'a congenital lack of hearing is not necessarily a harm' and that 'their lives are equally full' (Koch 2005: 124). People conduct their lives as they physically are, and this shapes their aspirations and social interactions so that in the end questions concerning the harmfulness or benefit of particular inborn conditions become virtually meaningless (Koch 2001: 373). Being deaf or lacking the tip of one's little finger is an integral part of who one is, not an emergency in need of medical attention.

Going beyond the question of harm, many people have argued that their physical conditions, described by others as disabilities, have actually been a positive force in their lives, individually and socially. Physicist Stephen Hawking has Amyotrophic Lateral Sclerosis which has gradually led to near-complete paralysis, but his contention is that this has actually been helpful for his academic career by making his style of writing economic and concise (Hawking 1993: 167). Many others have reported that their physical dependencies have been more than compensated for by 'an increased richness in interpersonal relations' (Koch 2001: 373, cf. 2000). And where an actual community of physically distinctive individuals exists, its culture and values should command the same respect as the culture and values of other majority and minority groups. This seems to be exemplified by the environment in which Sharon Duchesneau and Candace McCullough work and live with their children – Gallaudet University in Washington, DC, with most of the staff deaf and the majority of staff and students living in the vicinity (Mundy 2002; Parker 2007: 279).

The Social View does not deny that disabilities (as defined by the advocates of this View) can be, and often are, harmful. The harm is not, however, caused directly or necessarily by the difference or impairment individuals live with. It is caused by the attitudes of people without the difference or impairment and by the ensuing poor recognition of the needs of those with particular conditions. While differences are inevitable and morally neutral, disabilities are social constructs which harm individuals and groups to whom they are assigned (Vehmas 2004). The way to alleviate the situation is to focus on societal reactions and support systems, not on medically defined variations in individuals. Not hearing can be simply a condition, while deafness can be a culture, if allowed to be one, and a disability, if forced to be one.

The strength of the moral case for the Social View will be revisited in the eighth section below.

The case for legal permissiveness

Despite the disagreement at the moral level, defenders of the opposing models of disability potentially agree on the value of legal neutrality when it comes to selecting 'deaf embryos'. The agreement is an uneasy one, as I will further elaborate in the ninth section, but it is conceptually defensible.

The consequentialist advocates of the Medical View state strongly and repeatedly that what they say about the morality of selecting 'deaf embryos' should not be transformed into legal prohibitions or regulations. Harris (2000: 96, 100), while insisting that it is wrong to bring avoidable suffering into the world, is also adamant in declaring that parental choices should be respected as long as the resulting children can be expected to have at least a minimally decent life ahead of them. Unless the lives of individuals are so miserable that they would not on any account be worth leading, the individuals themselves are not harmed by bringing them into existence. According to Harris, 'most disabilities fall far short of the high standard of awfulness required to judge a life to be not worth living', which is why he professes to have 'consistently distinguished reasons for avoiding producing new disabled individuals from enforcement, regulation or prevention' (2000: 100) and 'always stoutly upheld the principle of reproductive freedom or reproductive autonomy' (ibid.: 96).

Another consequentialist champion of the Medical View, Julian Savulescu (2002: 772–773), explores the matter in some detail and supports reproductive freedom by quoting the nineteenth-century liberal utilitarianism of John Stuart Mill. In his theory, Mill (1859) argued that people should be allowed to experiment with different, even conflicting, practices and ideas, because this is the only way to prevent state oppression and eventually to find reasonable and mutually acceptable modes of living. If views which turn out to be right are suppressed, they may never be discovered by society as a whole. And if views which turn out to be wrong are suppressed, the right views can be accepted for the wrong reasons, and consequently applied incorrectly to changing situations in the future. This is why freedom of thought and action should prevail unless harm is inflicted on non-consenting others, individually or socially. Savulescu sees this as a sufficient foundation for parental autonomy in the context of most disabilities. Like Harris, he contends that individuals born with disabilities are not usually harmed by those who have produced them. And although he recognises the possibility that society could be economically hurt by an over-abundance of people with special needs, he is confident that this is not a serious concern, as 'it is unlikely that many people would make a selection for disability' (Savulescu 2002: 773). In all, although he believes that 'deafness ... is bad', he also believes that his 'value judgment should not be imposed on couples who must bear and rear the child' (ibid.: 772).

Those who hold the Social View may have difficulties with the general idea of reproductive autonomy, and I will return to these in the penultimate section. But in the specific case of deaf parents trying to have deaf offspring, the option of being legally required to do what others see as fit should not seem too attractive. After describing his own minor physical limitations, Koch (2001: 373), for instance, goes on to say that were '[his] partner currently pregnant and given the choice of a fetus with [his] genetic pattern or one that was "normal", [he] would likely choose the former'. And Sharon Duchesneau and Candace McCullough certainly 'wanted to increase [their] chances of having a baby who is deaf' seriously enough not to take an institutional 'no' for an answer: before soliciting the help of their deaf friend they had been turned down by the local sperm bank with a policy of excluding congenitally deaf donors (Mundy 2002). Choices such as these can only be accommodated by a legal permission to select 'deaf embryos'.

The instability of the situation

The academic debate described in the preceding sections shows that ethical opinion in the field is divided. Some insist that selecting 'deaf embryos' would be the moral equivalent of deliberately harming an innocent child; others counter that preventing that choice is the mark of an uncaring and discriminatory society. Attempts to reconcile the conflict have failed so far, and there is no reason to assume that similar endeavours will be more successful in the future (e.g. Reindal 2000; Harris 2000, 2001; Koch 2001, 2005; Savulescu 2002; Levy 2002; Anstey 2002; Häyry 2004a, 2004b; Singer 2005; Parker 2007).

Differences of opinion are, of course, common in real-life ethical discussions, and there are at least two ways of dealing with them. The first is to show that one of the competing views is self-evidently superior to all the others. I will demonstrate in the next two sections that this is not feasible in our current context, because both main views can be comprehensively challenged, even without using the premises employed by the competing camps. The second is to admit the disagreement and try to find practical compromises to the issue. In the concluding sections of the chapter I will explain why and how I would favour this route.

The moral case for the Medical View reconsidered

The defences given for the Medical View by John Harris are by no means unassailable. On closer examination, his 'medical ethics' view collapses into the consequentialist approach, and this, in its turn, logically implies a judgment that Harris consistently and vehemently denies.

The medical ethics, or 'do no harm', line assumes that a variety of different practices are morally on a par. These include the deafening of a hearing child, letting a child lose its hearing, not curing a deaf child, and selecting a 'deaf embryo'. The problem is that these practices are different in many respects that ethicists have seen as important. Some of them involve acts while others involve omissions (cf. Takala 2007). The intention of deafening the hearing child is presumably to harm the child, while selecting the 'deaf embryo' is meant to benefit the future individual (Mundy 2002). In the first cases a child already exists when the choice is made, but in the PGD case this is not true (Häyry 2004b). Some of these distinctions may be morally insignificant, but their presence suffices to cast doubt on the purely intuitive reaction expressed by Harris. Apart from his personal view, however, the only similarity between the four scenarios seems to be that they all result in someone being deaf. This is probably a relevant consideration, but it is markedly outcome-based, which means that the 'do no harm' appeal turns out to be just a variant of the more general consequentialist case.

This interim conclusion is quite possibly fatal to Harris's justification of the Medical View. If our moral duty, and our only moral duty, is to make the world as good as possible *and* if we have a moral duty not to have deaf children, then, by logical implication, deaf individuals make the world worse than hearing individuals. The world would be a better place without them. It would be better if they did not exist. We have a duty to see to it that they do not exist in future. Whichever way the sentence is twisted, it sounds discriminatory and callous. This is presumably why consequentialists are at pains to disown the view expressed by it. Harris (2001: 386, cf. 1992: 72–73), for instance, argues that although he would not like to lose one of his hands, he would not by losing a hand 'become less morally important, less valuable in … the "existential sense", more dispensable or more disposable'. According to him, 'to have a rational preference not to be disabled is not the same as having a rational preference for the non-disabled as persons'.

Other defenders of outcome-based ethics have made similar points and claimed that they see individuals with disabilities as equal persons with full rights

(Singer 2005: 133). But I do not see how they can escape the Callous Judgment. 'Hearing embryos' ought to be selected, because the resulting state of affairs would be better than if 'deaf embryos' are selected. This is due to the fact that deafness is a harmed condition which detracts value from a normal (hearing) life. Hence, a hearing life is better and a deaf life is worse. And since this judgment cannot be avoided in the consequentialist analysis provided by Harris, his defence of the Medical View is self-contradictory and must be rejected.

The moral case for the Social View reconsidered

The Social View does not have the internal logical problems that the Medical View suffers from, but it, too, can be challenged on at least three different grounds. Two of these have to do with the social and individual welfare of the eventual child, and the third is a plea for fairness and efficiency in providing for unavoidable as opposed to optional special needs. (A number of other concerns have been aired by the consequentialist defenders of the Medical View, but I have forgone these here because their credibility depends on the Medical View's already contested moral justification.)

The first objection questions, on a factual level, the idea of a deaf culture as the primary basis for personal identity. Defenders of the Social View argue that the children of deaf parents will have the best possible lives when they are members of a community which consists mainly of deaf people and in which the primary means of communication is sign language. Hearing would be an obstacle for their development, and it should not be favoured or pursued. While this can be true in principle and while the idea may just be workable in relatively established deaf environments such as at Gallaudet University and its neighbourhood, it is probably not practicable in many other contexts. Deaf communities are enveloped by homogenising wider societies, and their continued existence, as with the continued existence of any minority or majority culture, is always under potential threat. But if communities are not stable over time, they cannot be expected to guarantee their young the identity-building packages that are, according to the Social View itself, required for the best life as a deaf person. This leaves room for at least practical doubts about selecting 'deaf embryos' as a way to secure optimal lives for the children of deaf parents.

The second objection concentrates on the welfare of the individual regardless of the attitudes and actions of the surrounding community. Deafness in and by itself does not make a person generally unhealthy or less likely to contribute positively to the endeavours of the wider society. Recognition and support can replace the lack of hearing in dealings and communication with those who are not deaf. However, if intelligible contact with others is important for human flourishing, there is a catch here. It is that similar comments can be extended, separately, to sight and touch – two other main channels through which we interact with each other and with the world. We can, no doubt, live good lives without one or even two of these. But if for any reason we lose all three, we are, in the absence of telepathy or some fantastic new technology, well and truly isolated. Parents who do not want to gamble on the well-being of their children might want to consider even such improbable turns of events when they make their reproductive choices. Making children begin their lives without one of the three main instruments of communication inevitably increases the (marginal but existing) chance that they might, later in life, become totally cut off from others.[2]

The third objection raises questions about fairness and efficiency in the allocation of scarce resources. As one author comments, 'people might find it hard to accept that ... deaf people might prefer to have deaf children and then request society's support in order to be able to meet their children's special needs' (Munthe 1999: 239).[3] One reason for this possible reaction is that people themselves and their loved ones have needs, 'special' and not, and they are worried that these will be ignored in order to meet purely optional and superfluous claims created by parents who try to make copies of themselves. The latter part of this concern does not seem to be justified in the case of Sharon Duchesneau and Candace McCullough, for whom, reportedly, the future child's welfare as a part of their family was paramount (Mundy 2002). But this still leaves intact the comparison of optional and inevitable needs. If there is a limited amount of resources for 'special needs', then producing a child who is less likely to have them liberates resources to cater for already extant needs. And, other things being equal, a deaf child's likelihood to require societal adjustments is greater than a hearing child's probability of needing them. My logic in claiming this is the following. As long as lack of hearing requires adjustments from society, the deaf child's likelihood of having special needs is 100 per cent. If there are no other differences in health conditions or family circumstances, a hearing child's likelihood of having these special needs is less than 100 per cent – it is not zero, though, as the child could become deaf later. Whatever other needs individuals may have, these are in this calculation, by hypothesis, equally likely and equally extensive. I have also assumed that the potential contributions to society of deaf and hearing individuals are equal. Is it justifiable, then, to jeopardise the need satisfaction of people who do or will exist anyway for the sake of reproductive or communitarian wish-fulfilment?

Towards a Non-Directive Compromise

Since the moral cases for the Medical and Social Views are both convincing to their supporters, and since both can be plausibly challenged by third parties, it is improbable that the question of selecting 'deaf embryos' can be satisfactorily solved by claiming that one or the other case is universally valid and should therefore be accepted. This is why I believe that the solution is to admit that the practice is genuinely morally contested and to proceed to find other grounds for a palatable deal. The location of my suggested Non-Directive Compromise is presented schematically in Table 10.2.

My case for this Non-Directive Compromise can be outlined as follows. As I have described in the fifth section, even scholars who disagree on the moral status of selecting 'deaf embryos' can potentially agree on the permissive legal stand that should be taken in the matter. This is a welcome agreement, if non-

Table 10.2 The Non-Directive Compromise

Selecting the 'deaf embryos' is / should be			
↓ / →	**legally prohibited**	**legally permitted**	**legally required**
morally wrong	Medical View ⇦		
morally contested		Non-Directive Compromise	
morally right			⇨ Social View

directiveness is valued in parental counselling – and I think it should be. Neither the Medical View nor the Social View can, however, unequivocally support the permissive line, because in both models the underlying moral convictions create strong tensions towards a more rigid legislative stance. The full recognition of the moral contestedness of the practice can best lead to the desired and desirable leniency in legal terms.

The issue of the proper role of non-directiveness in genetic counselling is an unresolved one, mainly because definitions abound; many different types of genetic information are discussed simultaneously; and several authors reasonably doubt the clinicians' ability to provide neutral advice in matters in which their own minds are already made up (e.g. Suter 1998; Elwyn *et al.* 2000; Oduncu 2002). My notion here is that parental counselling is non-directive if and only if the healthcare practitioner does not intentionally or unintentionally persuade potential parents into making choices favoured by the practitioner. The emphasis in this kind of interaction is on the 'wisdom of the process', not on the 'wisdom of the decision' as seen by health professionals or authorities (Elwyn *et al.* 2000: 135).

One way to illustrate the value of non-directiveness in selecting 'deaf' or 'hearing' embryos is to consider it pragmatically in the context of political uncertainty. While advocates of the Medical and Social Views would prefer a situation in which their own kind of directiveness rules in genetic counselling, they cannot be sure that this is realistically achievable. To avoid the worst outcome, which is directiveness as defined by the opposition, it might be prudent for both parties to forgo attempts at control and to settle for the 'second best' alternative, which is non-directiveness (cf. Häyry 1991: 106–107). If it is too much to ask that individual practitioners could be value-neutral or present the cases for both sides, then teams of counsellors should perhaps be set up to explain to would-be parents the conflicting views on the matter. However the practicalities were arranged, unquestioned neutrality and permissiveness would be required at the level of the law. But this is a requirement that neither of the warring parties can confidently be trusted to meet.

As presented in Table 10.2, the Medical View has an intrinsic tendency to slide towards the restrictive direction. The main defence of legal permissiveness within the model's consequentialist variant is that social experiments should be allowed as long as they do not harm non-consenting individuals or communities. But it is far from clear that a lenient legislative line on selecting 'deaf embryos' would honour the stated caveat. If disabilities are harmed conditions and if deafness is a disability, the practice would allow the creation of future individuals in harmed conditions, which has a definite ring of allowing the production of future harm. This impression is fortified by Savulescu's (2002: 773) contention that the 'wrong' choices can and should be allowed only because so few parents would probably make them. What if many parents decided on conditions that consequentialists define as disabilities? By the logic of Savulescu's argument, this would call for legal prohibitions.

In a similar manner, the Social View is inclined to move towards the other legislative extreme. This inclination manifests itself, in our current context, indirectly. Champions of the model often see the general principle of parental freedom as an individualistic ploy that covers the rise of what they consider a new and frightening form of eugenics (Reindal 2000; Koch 2005). Governments no longer prevent the reproduction of 'unfit' citizens or families (on the 'old eugenics, see e.g. Buchanan *et al.* 2001), but under the cloak of individual autonomy and the freedom of the health market people are led to believe that all available genetic tests should be employed to prevent unwanted hereditary conditions. Since the situation is, so the argument goes, inherently coercive and detrimental to the interests of people with disabilities, parents should not be encouraged to make use of genetic testing. Yet this is exactly what legal leniency invites them to do, and this is why it should not be condoned. Parents should not be allowed to choose children without specific conditions like the ones probably leading to lack of hearing. Indirectly this means that in some situations people are legally required to choose the 'deaf embryos'. When the probability of deafness is very high to begin with, and PGD and ES are banned, the likeliest outcome is that the potential parents are forced by law to have deaf children if they want to have children at all.

The Non-Directive Compromise

The starting point of the Non-Directive Compromise is that the moral reasons for and against selecting 'deaf embryos', different as they are, have roughly equal weight, which means that the practice is genuinely morally contested. Since honest genetic counselling should reflect this situation, it cannot favour either the Medical View or the Social View. Rather than avoiding the ethical issues, however, comprehensive and honest counselling should convey the main thrust of both models to the potential parents. Instead of striving for artificial neutrality, the advice given can be 'multi-directive': in the interest of the 'wisdom of the process', two practitioners could try to make equally strong cases for the opposing views. The process itself could then ideally become non-directive in the sense that I defended in the previous section.

The Non-Directive Compromise is compatible with legal permissiveness regardless of the approach taken to the relationship between law and morality in the second section above. Natural law theorists would expect legislators to prohibit serious and unmistakable moral wrongs, but selecting 'deaf embryos' cannot be counted among these. Legal positivists need to see that the law has, by following its own historical logic, reached the permissive conclusion, which in many countries it has. And liberals require, and seem to be satisfied, that no serious harm is inflicted on innocent third parties.

Acceptance of the moral contestedness of selecting 'deaf embryos' strongly suggests the Non-Directive Compromise, and the legal permissiveness that goes with it appears to be supportable from most points of view. This is why I believe that the Non-Directive Compromise should be assumed.

Acknowledgement

This chapter was produced as a part of the project *Ethical and Social Aspects of Bioinformatics* (ESABI), financed from 2004–2007 by the Academy of Finland (SA 105139).

Notes

1 In the passage marked with [...] Harris continues that the chosen individual should 'have the best possible chance of a long and healthy life and the best possible chance of contributing positively to the world it will inhabit'. I have omitted this rhetorical addition because deafness and missing fingertips do not, as far as I know, have any direct or inevitable impact on longevity, general health or contribution to society.
2 This can be countered by saying that reproduction would become impossible if very small risks like these were taken into account in decisions to have children. Whether or not they should, and what the implications would be, see Häyry (2004c, 2005).
3 This citation does not, by the way, necessarily reflect the views of the author – Munthe is simply reporting what people in general could think about parents who do not want to use genetic testing to exclude the possibility of congenital deafness.

Bibliography

Anstey, K. W. (2002) 'Are Attempts to Have Impaired Children Justifiable?', *Journal of Medical Ethics*, 28: 286–8.
Baruch, S., Kaufman, D. and Hudson, K. L. (2006) 'Genetic Testing of Embryos: Practices and Perspectives of US In Vitro Fertilisation Clinics', *Fertility and Sterility,* in press.
Buchanan, A., Brock, D. W., Daniels, N. and Wikler, D. (2001) *From Chance to Choice: Genetics and Justice*, Cambridge: Cambridge University Press.
Elwyn, G., Gray, J. and Clarke, A. (2000) 'Shared Decision Making and Non-Directiveness in Genetic Counselling', *Journal of Medical Genetics*, 37: 135–8.
Gillon, R. (1985) *Philosophical Medical Ethics*, Chichester: John Wiley and Sons.
Hare, R. M. (1976) 'Survival of the Weakest', in S. Gorovitz (ed.), *Moral Problems in Medicine*, Englewood Cliffs, NJ: Prentice-Hall.
Harris, J. (1992) *Wonderwoman and Superman: The Ethics of Human Biotechnology*, Oxford: Oxford University Press.
—— (2000) 'Is There a Coherent Social Conception of Disability?', *Journal of Medical Ethics*, 26: 95–100.
—— (2001) 'One Principle and Three Fallacies of Disability Studies', *Journal of Medical Ethics*, 27: 383–7.
—— (2007) *Enhancing Evolution: The Ethical Case for Making Better People*, Princeton, NJ: Princeton University Press.

Hawking, S. (1993) *Black Holes and Baby Universes*, New York: Bantam Books.

Häyry, H. (1991) *The Limits of Medical Paternalism*, London and New York: Routledge.

—— (1994) *Liberal Utilitarianism and Applied Ethics*, London and New York: Routledge.

—— (1999) 'What the Fox Would Have Said, Had He Been a Hedgehog: on the Methodology and Normative Approach of John Harris's Wonderwoman and Superman', in V. Launis, J. Pietarinen and J. Räikkä (eds), *Genes and Morality: New Essays*, Amsterdam and Atlanta, GA: Rodopi.

—— (2004a) 'If You Must Make Babies, Then at Least Make the Best Babies You Can?', *Human Fertility*, 7: 105–12.

—— (2004b) 'There Is a Difference Between Selecting a Deaf Embryo and Deafening a Hearing Child', *Journal of Medical Ethics*, 30: 510–12.

—— (2004c) 'A Rational Cure for Pre-Reproductive Stress Syndrome', *Journal of Medical Ethics*, 30: 377–8.

—— (2005) 'The Rational Cure for Prereproductive Stress Syndrome Revisited', *Journal of Medical Ethics*, 31: 606–7.

—— (2007) 'Utilitarianism and Bioethics', in R. E. Ashcroft, A. Dawson, H. Draper and J. R. McMillan (eds), *Principles of Health Care Ethics*, 2nd edn, Chichester: John Wiley and Sons.

Koch, T. (2000) 'Life Quality Vs the "Quality of Life": Assumptions Underlying Prospective Quality of Life Instruments in Health Care Planning', *Social Science and Medicine*, 51: 419–28.

—— (2001) 'Disability and Difference: Balancing Social and Physical Constructions', *Journal of Medical Ethics*, 27: 370–6.

—— (2005) 'The Ideology of Normalcy: The Ethics of Difference', *Journal of Disability Policy Studies*, 16: 123–9.

Levy, N. (2002) 'Deafness, Culture, and Choice', *Journal of Medical Ethics*, 28: 284–5.

Mill, J. S. (1859) *On Liberty*, reprinted in J. S. Mill, *On Liberty and The Subjection of Women*, Ware: Wordsworth, 1996.

Mundy, L. (2002) 'A World of Their Own', *Washington Post*, 31 March, p. W22.

Munthe, C. (1999) *Pure Selection: The Ethics of Preimplantation Genetic Diagnosis and Choosing Children without Abortion*, Gothenburg: Acta Universitatis Gothoburgensis.

Oduncu, F. S. (2002) 'The Role of Non-Directiveness in Genetic Counseling', *Medicine, Health Care and Philosophy*, 5: 53–63.

Parker, M. (2007) 'The Best Possible Child', *Journal of Medical Ethics*, 33: 279–83.

Reindal, S. M. (2000) 'Disability, Gene Therapy and Eugenics: A Challenge to John Harris', *Journal of Medical Ethics*, 26: 89–94.

Robertson, J. A. (2003) 'Extending Preimplantation Genetic Diagnosis: The Ethical Debate', *Human Reproduction*, 18: 465–71.

Savulescu, J. (2001) 'Procreative Beneficence: Why We Should Select the Best Children', *Bioethics*, 15: 413–26.

—— (2002) 'Deaf Lesbians, "Designer Disability," and the Future of Medicine', *British Medical Journal*, 325: 771–3.

Singer, P. (2005) 'Ethics and Disability: A Response to Koch', *Journal of Disability Policy Studies*, 16: 130–3.

Spriggs, M. (2002) 'Lesbian Couple Create a Child Who Is Deaf Like Them', *Journal of Medical Ethics*, 28: 283.

Suter, S. M. (1998) 'Value Neutrality and Nondirectiveness: Comments on "Future Directions in Genetic Counseling"', *Kennedy Institute of Ethics Journal*, 8: 161–3.

Takala, T. (2003) 'Utilitarianism Shot Down by Its Own Men', *Cambridge Quarterly of Healthcare Ethics*, 12: 447–54.

—— (2007) 'Acts and Omissions', in R. E. Ashcroft, A. Dawson, H. Draper and J. R. McMillan (eds), *Principles of Health Care Ethics*, 2nd edn, Chichester: John Wiley and Sons.

Vehmas, S. (2004) 'Ethical Analysis of the Concept of Disability', *Mental Retardation*, 42: 209–22.

Vehmas, S. and Mäkelä, P. (2008) 'A Realist Account of the Ontology of Impairment', *Journal of Medical Ethics*, 34: 93–5.

11 The role of medical experts in shaping disability law

Lindsey Brown

Introduction

Law impacts significantly on disabled people. Furthermore there is an intrinsic connection between law and societal values so when a particular set of values or conceptual model is enshrined in law, its coercive effect may stigmatise disabled people. It is important, therefore, to explore the ways in which lawmakers frame disability issues. This chapter aims to explore the relationship between how 'disability' is perceived in the United Kingdom (UK) and the laws resulting from those attitudes. Two key UK lawmakers are the legislature (parliament) and the judiciary (courts) (Holland and Webb 2006). Laws stemming from parliament take the form of statutes and regulations;[1] laws are made by courts through the reasoning adopted in cases (Holland and Webb 2006).[2] This chapter focuses on judge-made law (case law) in the context of what have become known as 'end-of-life' cases. It concentrates on three recent, controversial disputes that have been played out before the courts in England and Wales.[3] Through analysing the discourses employed by judges in these cases, this chapter seeks to demonstrate the almost imperceptible yet insidious impact of what may be called the 'medical model' of disability. Its profound and often detrimental influence stems, in part, from judges' reliance on medical professionals as 'experts' in these cases.

Many terms are used by the media, health professionals, courts and parliament to describe the judgements and assumptions made about disability and disabled people. Phrases such as 'lives not worth living', 'best interests', 'intolerability' and 'welfare' appear frequently. All such terms involve judgements about the 'quality of life' of individuals. Consequently, unpacking them is important when discussing disability. Furthermore, such quality of life (QL) judgements affect the law in the field of health care for disabled people. QL instruments are used in relation to both individual decisions as well as to strategic health planning. The result has been an increasing reliance in health-care planning, and medical decision making generally, on quantitative and prospective, health-related QL instruments (Frisch 1994; Testa and Nackley 1994). The most infamous of QL instruments are quality adjusted life years (QALYS) which represent medico-legal orthodoxy in the matter of health-care allocation.

Different areas of law use different terms to assess the individuals' QL. 'Best interests' decision-making is one of the guises of QL judgements used most often by UK judges. Accordingly, it forms the focus of this chapter. Whilst QL itself is a much contested term in academic literature, in particular in philosophy (e.g., Walter and Shannon 1990) and social science (e.g., Wasserman *et al.* 2005), there remains little agreement as to whether or not QL should be assessed objectively (objective measures of functioning and participation) or subjectively (based on the patient's own judgements and feelings) (Wasserman *et al.* 2005). It is perhaps surprising that the use of QL as the correct approach for decision-making in health-care law cases has not been widely debated since *Bland*,[4] when the courts expressed the view that it may be in the 'best interests' of patients who are in a 'persistent vegeta-tive state' to be permitted to die.[5] Thus, the focus has been on how 'meaningful' life is for the patient – i.e., a QL approach. Judgements based on the 'best interests' of the incapacitated patient have become commonplace and widely accepted, whilst the utility of 'best interests' as a term is rarely scrutinised.

The focus of much of the discussion in this chapter will be on the three cases of Charlotte Wyatt,[6] Leslie Burke,[7] and MB.[8] *Wyatt*, *Burke* and *MB* are all recent, controversial end-of-life cases that attracted substantial media interest involving a patient or their family trying to insist on specific treatments, whilst the health-care trusts treating them wish to withdraw or to withhold such treatments.[9] Tex-tual analysis of the various judgements in these cases clearly demonstrates the attitudes held by lawmakers when assessing the QL of disabled people.

The utility of the traditional models described in disability theory is often debated. Whilst recent writings (e.g., Shakespeare 2006) have suggested that the traditional models of disability should be abandoned, this chapter will continue to refer to both medical and social models in order to illustrate the approaches taken by the judiciary in their reasoning of these cases. The models of disabil-ity continue to provide a vocabulary well known and understood. The continued reliance of the courts upon and acceptance of a medical perspective in this these cases demonstrate that UK lawmakers are not inclined to question – let alone to contradict – the influence of the medical model of disability.

The cases

Before turning to the theoretical framework, it is essential to briefly outline the three selected cases. Charlotte Wyatt was born after twenty-six weeks' gesta-tion in 2003 with serious heart and lung problems. Doctors at her hospital trust believed that, if she stopped breathing, they should not revive her, as her QL would be too poor and dominated by pain. But her parents wanted her to be given a tracheostomy. The High Court judge, Mr Justice Hedley (hereafter referred to as Hedley J) found in favour of the NHS Trust.[10] Charlotte's parents have brought the case back to court several times as she continues to survive and, in their opinion, develop.[11] Yet, Hedley J has refused to change his opinion. Part of the case also was heard in the Court of Appeal which, again, found in favour of the NHS Trust.[12]

Leslie Burke, who has a degenerative brain condition, took the General Medical Council (GMC) to court over their guidance on artificial nutrition and hydration (ANH) at the end of life. He wanted to stop doctors being able to withdraw ANH from him when he could no longer speak. Initially, Mr Justice Munby (hereafter referred to as Munby J) in the High Court found that the GMC guidelines were inadequate.[13] However, this was overruled by the Court of Appeal who found that the application for judicial review of the GMC's rules was unnecessary because the rules and the law which they summarised protected him adequately.[14] When Burke's application for permission to appeal to the House of Lords was refused, he took his case to the European Court of Human Rights (ECtHR).[15] The ECtHR declined his application, which sought effectively to overturn the Court of Appeal's ruling that it might be lawful for doctors to withdraw ANH once Mr Burke lost competence to determine his own best interests.

The parties in *MB* were the parents of a baby with severe spinal muscular atrophy and the health-care trust treating him.[16] The NHS Trust sought permission to withdraw ventilation, whilst MB's parents wanted the doctors to perform a tracheostomy. The doctors considered that MB's QL was so low, and the burdens of living for him so great, that it was unethical and unlawful to continue to keep him alive artificially. Conversely, MB's parents believed that he had some QL: in particular, that he gained pleasure from his family, music, DVDs and television. Mr Justice Holman (hereafter referred to as Holman J) decided in favour of the parents, insofar as he refused the NHS Trust permission to withdraw ventilation. But he would not order the doctors to perform a tracheostomy. This was the first time that a court had been asked to approve, against the will of the parents, the withdrawal of life support from a child with 'sensory awareness, assumed normal cognition and no reliable evidence of brain damage' (Foster 2006a).

Theoretical frames for exploring these cases

Disability can be placed within a number of different frames which have the power to make us see disability in one way rather than another. How disability is framed by lawmakers directly influences the laws that they produce. Commentators suggest that the dominant culture tends to reflect the interests of those within particular social groups who have the power to define situations and the necessary resources to ensure that their own definitions are accepted as true e.g., Saraga 1998). While space precludes detailed consideration of these ideas here, they serve as a possible explanation for the dominance of the medical model of disability within UK law and medicine. The argument here is that, as a result of the traditional hegemony of medicine, 'disability' has been defined within an individualised medical model. Medicine, despite recent bad press, is still held in high esteem within UK society (Goble 2003: 46). Clinical definitions have their basis in the authority that attaches to medicine as carried out by medical specialists (Altman 2001: 99). Within the scope of this chapter, this theoretical backdrop helps both to illuminate and explain how and why UK courts implicitly accept doctors' medical evidence as being the most appropriate way to formulate QL judgements in relation to disabled people. Yet, this is problematic – not least, because evidence strongly suggests that doctors judge disabled people's QL differently from how they judge their own lives.

Medical doctors' views of the quality of life of disabled people

Much research suggests that doctors' QL judgements characteristically are based on the limited perspective of medical diagnosis and prognosis rather than on any fuller exploration or understanding of patients' lives. Consequently, they have limited value. Doctors usually are not experts themselves in living with disabilities, and are not necessarily well informed about everyday life experiences of disabled people.[17] Asch, for example, describes how doctors substitute an ill-formed social judgement about disability for a medical one (Asch 1988: 77–87). Doctors receive little or no education about the realities of living with disability;[18] nor does their training qualify them to judge the social elements of people's lives. Yet, properly undertaken QL assessments should not solely rely on a doctor's *medical* opinion of whether treatment should be given or withdrawn, but also on the patient's *social welfare.* Whilst doctors can claim to have medical expertise, they cannot claim any special expertise in assessing the many non-medical matters which also should underpin decisions about what is in the patient's best interests. Doctors' opinions may well stem, therefore, from a backdrop of negative images and poorly informed assumptions about 'intolerable' suffering, unacceptable dependence on others, or that particular disabilities make life 'not worth living'.[19] Much of the disability-rights critique of doctors in this respect centres on their 'failures of imagination' (Parens and Asch 2000: 8) – i.e., their inability to imagine that disabled people might lead lives equally as valuable, rich and complex as their own. Doctors may only see disabled people as 'patients' in a consulting room, usually during health crises. Even physicians who regularly treat disabled people may have inaccurate impressions of such people's lives if they interact with them only in a medical setting (Andrews 2002: 104). Few doctors get to know their patients personally, or how they live their lives outside the consulting room. They may not necessarily have contact with disabled adults as equals and peers (Ward 2002: 194). Other health professionals, such as occupational therapists and district nurses, may have more expertise than doctors at knowing how impairments actually affect the QL of disabled people. Yet, because they do not go through such extensive medical training they are not seen as 'experts', and instead defer to doctors who manage patients' care.[20]

It is worth noting that not only may doctors not necessarily review the situation comprehensively; there is evidence that they also make objectively demonstrable errors in both diagnosis and prognosis. In his work on the 'persistent vegetative state', Andrews demonstrates that of forty patients referred as being in the vegetative state, seventeen (43 per cent) were considered as having been misdiagnosed. In fact many of the patients misdiagnosed in this way were actually blind or had severe visual impairment (Andrews 1996). Many declarations by medics of diagnosis or prognosis are interpretations, yet in the courts are treated as fact.[21]

A great deal of evidence illustrates the considerable variance between the views of disabled people and physicians on QL (e.g., Rothwell *et al.* 1997). Physicians tend to underestimate the QL of disabled people. For example, in one study 82 per cent of doctors surveyed indicated that their QL would be relatively low if they had quadriplegia. In contrast, 80 per cent of people with quadriplegia rated the quality of their lives as 'pretty good' (Gallagher 1995). In another study, only 18 per cent of emergency-room professionals surveyed believed that traumatic spinal-cord injury patients could achieve an acceptable life quality; whereas 92 per cent of those who had survived spinal-cord injury (resulting in long-term disability) reported positive life valuations (Gerhart *et al.* 1994). Put simply, surrogate judgements often do not accurately reflect patients' own perceptions or preferences (Addington-Hall and Kalra 2001). As Cella states, 'The external determination of a diminished or unacceptable life is often not shared by the person whose life is being judged' (Cella 1992: 9). QL assessments by 'normal', 'healthy' persons can reflect the prejudices, fears or concerns of the observer, not those of the person whose lived existence is being judged. Thus, 'it often happens that lives which observers consider of poor quality are lived quite satisfactorily by the one living that life' (Reinders 2000: 161). Furthermore, there is evidence to suggest that people who make advance directives change their preferences and their views when they are actually in the situation envisaged by their advance directive (Sehgal *et al.* 1992).

Case law analysis: four key themes

Returning now to the three end-of-life cases, close textual analysis reveals at least four key themes, which will be presented in the following order: (1) the role of doctors as 'experts'; (2) the medical profession's dominance over court proceedings; (3) how medical evidence goes unchallenged; and (4) the supposed 'objectiveness' of QL judgements.

Doctors as 'experts'

As previously argued, doctors may not be the best 'experts' in judging the QL of disabled people. Indeed, Kennedy has argued that the prevailing 'best interests' test protects medical power rather than patient welfare (Kennedy 1988: 395–6). This view is supported by Montgomery, who argues that 'the duty to give incompetent patients the care that is in their best interests is usually judged not against the judicial assessment of where those interests lie but that of the doctors looking after them' (2000: 164). Montgomery also observes that, because many cases do not go to court, 'the application of the best interests principle lies in the hands of health professionals rather than lawyers' (ibid.: 164). Even when cases do come to court, judges tend to focus simply on ensuring that the clinical judgements made are within the parameters of responsible professional decisions. Thus, in *Re J*[22] it was said that it would be an abuse of the court's powers to instruct a doctor to treat against her or his clinical judgement. It will become evident that this reasoning was followed in *Wyatt, Burke*, and, to some extent, in *MB*. Montgomery further claims that 'there is significant danger that best interests decision making could become little more than a mechanism for the imposition of prejudice' (2000: 166). This is a real concern to disabled people because prejudiced QL judgements could mean the withdrawal of treatment, services or life-saving equipment.

How the 'best interests' test is constructed is important. Whilst often stating that the best interests test is not solely medical, it will be shown that the judiciary then continue to consider only the medical evidence, thereby undermining their rhetoric. It is therefore predictable that doctors are seen as suitable 'experts' to make QL judgements. However, as already argued, QL judgements properly should include social elements, and medics are not necessarily experts in disability issues. Furthermore, they typically take a view of disability that is grounded in the medical model.

There is much to be said for Munby J's approach to the issue of expertise in assessing best interests in the *Burke* case. As he suggested:

> The doctor's duty is not merely to act in accordance with a responsible and competent body of relevant professional opinion: his duty is to act in accordance with the patient's *best* interests ... The decisions as to what is in fact in the patient's best interests is not for the doctor: it is for the patient, if competent, or if the patient is incompetent and the matter comes to court, for the judge.[23]

Munby J's dictum aims to balance the power relationship between doctor and patient. Each has a breadth of knowledge and experience not available to the other. His approach considers the knowledge base of both patient and doctor to be of equal merit, such that neither should take precedence over the other as a matter of course. Moreover, in the final analysis, his decision suggests that the patient's wish to receive life-prolonging treatment should be met unless to do so would prolong an intolerable situation. Munby J seems to understand that doctors should not be asked, or be expected, to pass sole judgement over what is 'in the best interests' of a severely ill or disabled patient. Whilst doctors are clinical experts, they are not experts in deciding a more holistic concept of 'best interests'. Regretfully, it will be shown that the medical profession continue to dominate court proceedings and their evidence remains most influential.

The approach taken in *Re MB* was in contrast to Munby J's approach to expertise by defining respective roles for courts and for doctors. As Holman J tellingly observed:

> I wish to stress and make clear, however, that I myself am not concerned with any ethical issues which may surround this case ... The ethical decision whether actually to withdraw or withhold [life support] must be made by the doctors concerned. Judges are neither qualified to make, nor required, nor entitled to make ethical judgements or decisions.[24]

He seems to be saying that it was for doctors alone to decide the morality of withdrawing treatment from MB. Yet, were this correct, then there would have been no need for the case to come to court. The ethical decision simply would have been made by the doctors. Such an approach is deeply problematic, not least, because doctors will typically form their QL judgements based on medical model assumptions and perspectives.

The medical profession's dominance of court proceedings

In the *Wyatt* case, all the medical evidence submitted described how terrible Charlotte's QL was, and how she experienced only intolerable pain. It is clear on reading the High Court judgement that the judge relied heavily on this medical evidence to make his decision. Indeed, the medical evidence 'trumped' other evidence demonstrating that Charlotte could experience some QL. When looking at the judgement, the dominating influence of medical evidence becomes clear. From a judgement of twenty-two paragraphs,[25] ten were concerned with medical opinions.

In *MB*, a slew of doctors provided evidence: two as 'treating doctors',[26] eight more from the NHS Trust (part of the overall clinical team caring for MB, referred to as the 'trust doctors'),[27] and still others as expert witnesses.[28] The two 'treating doctors' provided detailed reports; the four 'expert witnesses' agreed a joint expert report;[29] and the 'trust doctors' each made statements. All the doctors' evidence agreed with that of the NHS Trust. Yet, the senior nurse of the intensive care unit also provided a statement, noting that there was disagreement among the nursing staff over MB's future treatment.[30] Despite the fact that some nurses disagreed with withdrawing MB's treatment, the judge concluded that, 'there is thus a very formidable body of medical evidence of very high quality in this case which is all, *without exception*, to the same effect'.[31]

Consideration of the medical evidence supplied by the NHS Trust and the 'expert witnesses' formed a large part of Holman J's judgement in *MB*. Yet, as already explained, apart from the senior nurse's statement (seemingly discounted by the judge), the doctors all concurred in their opinions. It is interesting to note that the 'trust doctors' (not including the 'treating doctors') all submitted identical witness statements, as all were in agreement with the 'treating doctors' about the correct course of action. Furthermore, the 'expert witnesses' all met to discuss their findings before submitting a joint expert report. In this way, it could be said that the court effectively was shut out of the decision-making process. The experts all agreed amongst themselves upon the 'correct' course of action; the court then had to rely on that body of opinion.

Holman J recognised that 'the views and opinions of both the doctors *and* the parents must be carefully considered'.[32] This implies that it is not just the medics who should provide insights into MB's QL. Yet, he then went on to discount MB's parents' opinions as they 'may, very understandably, be coloured by their own emotion or sentiment'.[33] Holman J reiterated how the parents failed to be objective by saying at another point that the mother was 'deluding herself'.[34] This is interesting as he qualifies his use of the opinions of parents, but offers no qualifications as to the use of doctors' opinions, thereby implying that doctors' opinions are more 'objective'.

Medical assessments should not be left unchallenged

As Sir Thomas Bingham MR said in *Frenchay Healthcare National Health Service Trust* v. *S*, 'It is, I think, important that there should not be a belief that what the doctor says is in the patient's best interest *is* in the patient's best interest.'[35] Yet traditionally, UK courts have merely relied on doctors' QL opinions.[36] How courts weigh medical evidence is of particular interest; especially when determining the facts of the case. In *Wyatt*, for example, it could be said that the judges selectively analysed the evidence before them, so that what appears to be factual description was, in reality, merely interpretation.[37] For example, the Court of Appeal seemed to ignore the evidence indicating an improvement in Charlotte's condition, focussing instead on the doctors' views of her 'intolerable' condition.

In the High Court, Hedley J stated that, 'after careful and anxious consideration, I find myself convinced by the majority of medical opinion'.[38] In fact, he seemed to have discounted all other evidence. Evidence presented from a home-visiting educational service for pre-school children recorded (*inter alia*) Charlotte as enjoying her bath; appearing to listen and respond to speech by looking at the speaker's face; smiling or turning her head and demonstrating some vision; and looking 'at surroundings (20 cms) when lying on her back'.[39] This evidence was supported by her guardian, who said: 'Charlotte can show what may be "enjoyment" of things now. She makes facial movements, opening her mouth and eyes a bit more, that might suggest she gains some pleasure, e.g. when she is being tickled.'[40] However, despite these improvements, the court constantly referred to there having been 'no change in her underlying clinical condition', such that the assessment of her QL and best interests had therefore not changed. This seems an extraordinary approach to take. For, surely, by indicating that Charlotte's QL had apparently improved, this evidence should have led to a reassessment of whether or not life-saving treatment was now in her best interests.

Once the court opted to take this approach, however, there was only one decision that could have been made. In accepting the doctors' views of the situation as comprehensive, and in finding that they were not making irresponsible decisions, the court was never going to find in favour of Charlotte's parents. Three elements combined to make the result inevitable: the 'trumping' effect of the medical evidence; the court's unwillingness to recognise any positive 'right' to treatment; and fear of undermining doctors or interfering with clinical decisions. This can be seen when the Court of Appeal stated: 'It is not the function of the court to be used as a general advice centre ... it is, in our view, not the function of the court to oversee the treatment plan for a gravely ill child. That function is for the doctors in consultation with the child's parents.'[41]

The most recent case of *MB* may demonstrate that progress is being made in this respect. In his judgement, Holman J made some critical comments about the medical evidence supplied. For example, he noted that all the statements from the 'trust doctors' were identical, all saying (*inter alia*) that MB 'already has an intolerably poor quality of life and this will only get worse'.[42] With reference to these statements, Holman J said, 'I do comment that within the common statement there is no reference to, or recognition of, any possible current pleasure or benefit to M from his life.'[43]

In this way, the judge recognised the limitations of the medical evidence. This was again evident when commenting on the 'balance sheets' detailing the benefits and burdens of continuing ventilation that the interested parties[44] were asked to submit. In relation to the NHS Trust's information, he said:

> I record, however, that even at the end of the hearing, the list ... on behalf of the Trust ... contains under the heading 'Benefit' only one item 'Preservation of life'. Whilst that may be said to be all embracing, it does not recognise or identify any specific benefit that M may be getting from his life, though the 'Disbenefits' are listed with considerable specific detail.[45]

Again, the judge implicitly recognised the subjective and selective nature of the medical evidence, which failed to acknowledge any social benefits to MB in remaining alive. By questioning the medical evidence, the judge believed that he was performing an objective assessment. The extent to which this was achieved will be analysed in the next section.

The objectiveness of QL assessments

The Court of Appeal in *Burke* suggested that a life lived with a condition that causes 'an extreme degree of pain, discomfort or indignity to a patient' should be considered not worth living, thereby absolving doctors from the positive duty to keep the patient alive.[46] Yet, all those terms are highly subjective and context-sensitive. People have different pain thresholds: what some might consider uncomfortable or undignified does not make life not worth living for others. As Asch comments, 'It is no more demeaning to obtain help in dressing or washing from a personal assistant than it is to get services from an auto mechanic, a plumber, or a computer technician' (2001: 313). Just because a person is unable to communicate or to articulate their views clearly, it does not mean that their life is not worth living. Many people with very severe intellectual impairments are able to experience and express pleasure and pain, show awareness of their surroundings and relationships, and demonstrate all the feelings associated with being a human subject (Shakespeare 1998: 665).

As Montgomery observes, 'once declared incompetent, patients become vulnerable to medical and judicial paternalism. The purpose of judicial scrutiny of decisions taken in the "best interests" of patients is to ensure that as objective a view as possible is taken' (Montgomery 2000: 178). Whilst in theory the courts' views are meant to be objective, in reality this is impossible. Inevitably, they will be influenced by cultural norms and values. On several occasions in *MB*, Holman

J reiterated the court's role in making a supposedly 'objective' assessment about MB's best interests. For example, he said his task, 'difficult enough in itself, is to decide, and only to decide, where the objective balance of the best interests of M lies'.[47] In an attempt to do this, he followed the Court of Appeal's guidance in *Wyatt* as to how to carry out a 'best interests' assessment:[48]

> The test is one of best interests, and the task of the court is to balance all the factors. The Court of Appeal have suggested that the best and safest way of reliably doing this is to draw up a list on which are specifically identified, on the one hand, the benefits or advantages and, on the other hand, the burdens or disadvantages of continuing or discontinuing the treatment in question.[49]

As already alluded to, it was for this reason that Holman J asked all interested parties to draw up their own balance sheets. As previously noted, he was unimpressed by the information provided by the NHS Trust. Yet, having completed this exercise, Holman J recognised the limitations in this approach, noting that, 'whilst it is a very helpful but relatively easy task to draw a list of benefits and burdens, there are still huge difficulties in striking the balance'. One of the principal difficulties he identified is making an 'overall appraisal of the weight to be attached to so many varied considerations which cannot be weighed "mathematically," and so arrive at the final balance and decision'.[50] Thus, it is impossible for courts or doctors to make purely objective assessments about someone's QL or what is in their best interests.[51] In particular, this is because most assessments made by the people in power rely on doctors' evidence.

Yet, there is recognition in *MB* that, despite a poor medical prognosis, there can still be benefits in life. For example, Holman J states:

> It is impossible to put a mathematical or any other value on the benefits. But they are precious and real and they are the benefits, and only benefits, that M was destined to gain from his life. I do not consider that from one day to the next all the routine discomfort, distress and pain that the doctors describe ... outweigh those benefits so that I can say that it is in his best interests that those benefits, and life itself, should immediately end. On the contrary, I positively consider that as his life does still have benefits, and is his life, it should be enabled to continue, subject to excluding the treatment I have identified.[52]

In this way, Holman J could be seen to have recognised the importance of resisting negative assumptions. By distinguishing *Re C*,[53] Holman J could be interpreted as trying to reject the medical model. For, had he looked only at the medical facts, as happened in *Re C*, he would have found in favour of the NHS Trust (because the evidence was so overwhelming). While Holman J did not go so far as to take a 'social model' approach to disability, he did at least seem to recognise some of the limitations of the medical model. In this regard, he recognised that doctors do not take into account anything outside the medical assessment. His judgement provides encouragement that, perhaps, UK lawmakers are beginning to appreciate that the medical model is not good enough as a basis on which to judge people's best interests, least of all in end-of-life situations.

The 'best interests' test (as it currently stands) is inadequate. It leaves far too many questions open, and needs further explanation. 'Best interests' often begs too many philosophical and theological questions to be confidently answered – and it is dangerously likely to be answered in a way which does not give the desirable (and legally mandatory) priority to the presumption in favour of continued life for disabled people (Foster 2006b). Furthermore, the test is currently assessed by medics utilising an approach that focuses on medical considerations without sufficient consideration of social elements.

Conclusions

This chapter has highlighted the courts' continued reluctance to acknowledge the social effects of disability when assessing QL. In part, this failure stems from judges' approach to considering disability, and the construction of the 'best interests' test that they choose to adopt. Whilst often stating that best interests is not purely medical, the judiciary continue to consider only the medical evidence, thereby effectively construing best interests as a medical test. As a result it is perhaps obvious that courts will regard doctors as appropriate 'experts' to provide the most cogent QL evidence. It is important that the judiciary consider the importance of the social elements of QL. As argued above, doctors are typically not qualified to assess these all-important social elements of disability. Moreover, generally speaking, their evaluations of the quality of disabled lives often contradict the views of disabled people themselves. Because of the close relationship between how disability is perceived and the laws that result, this continued dominance of a flawed approach dominating judicial thinking in this area ultimately leads to impoverished law. To improve the lives of disabled people, the negative assumptions and cultural values underlying QL assessments need to be exposed, unpacked and challenged. The analysis here suggests a wider construction of 'best interests' needs to be applied, such as that advocated by Munby J in *Burke*. There is a clear need to move away from a test that reflects only medical elements, and a need to empower patients when they are competent. Where patients are not competent, it is imperative that courts do not automatically accept or prefer doctors' views or assessments, and that best interests be approached from the patients' point of view.

Clearly, it is much better for disabled people if there is effective dialogue between health professionals, patients and their families. The 'partnership of care' approach (RCPCH 2004) should be utilised so that all parties are involved in decision-making. With the continued development of a multi-disciplinary care approach within the NHS, the courts should be more willing to consider evidence from health professionals other than medics who may have a valid contribution to make. However, there will be instances when parties cannot agree. It is imperative that when such cases come to court judges do not rebuke patients or their families for not agreeing with the doctors.[54] It is also important that judges recognise and accept that courts have a proper role to play in overseeing these decisions instead of abjuring responsibility, such as by hiding behind remarks that it is not for courts to make clinical[55] or ethical[56] decisions.

Ultimately, the courts are in an unenviable situation of trying to decide cases in which there is fundamental disagreement between the parties involved on patients' QL, and whether or not particular treatments are in patients' best interests. Historically, UK courts have tried to insist that they remain 'objective' in their deliberations. However, as shown above, QL judgements are often arbitrary and based on subjective preferences. Foster argues that the test of 'best interests' needs to be clarified by the courts. If the test is to be subjective, the person whose view is definitive needs to be identified; if the test is objective (as the judges currently claim it is), the criteria used in making the decision, along with the values which underpin the criteria, need to be extrapolated (Foster 2005). Currently the courts claim that they are making objective decisions; however, the way they apply this objective test is not clear, and therefore their judgements remain open to the criticism that instead they are making subjective decisions, the view of the courts being definitive. The key concern in the context of a disability-rights approach is that such judgements are made against a backdrop of prejudicial attitudes towards disability and the assumption that disability naturally leads to an impoverished QL. It is also impossible for the courts to remain objective when cases remain dominated by the medical profession and medical evidence. *MB* shows signs of potential progress in this respect, by questioning the doctors' evidence, and by recognising that MB had positive elements to his life that the doctors were not capable of assessing or taking into account. It is to be hoped that future courts will develop this approach even further.

Notes

1 Key legislation relevant to decision-making regarding the providing, withholding or withdrawing treatment includes the Children Act 1989 (when the patient is a child), the Human Rights Act 1998, and the Mental Capacity Act 2005 (when it comes into force).
2 This reasoning (the *ratio decidendi* – meaning the reason, or rationale, for the decision) becomes binding on courts of equal or lower status through the doctrine of binding precedent. When a case with similar issues or facts comes before a court subsequently, the court must follow the previous case.
3 Scotland and Northern Ireland have separate court systems and laws. However, for convenience the term 'UK' will be used.
4 *Airedale NHS Trust* v. *Bland* [1993] AC 789 (HL).
5 *Re H* [1998] 3 FCR 174; *Re D* [1998] 1 FCR 498; *Re R* [1996] 3 FCR 473. Some judges have argued that patients in PVS have no interests at all and so the best interests equation never enters the analysis.
6 *Portsmouth NHS Trust* v. *Wyatt* [2004] EWHC 2247 (Fam), [2005] 1 FLR 21 (hereafter *Wyatt I*); *Portsmouth Hospitals NHS Trust* v. *Wyatt* [2005] EWHC 117 (Fam) (hereafter *Wyatt II*); *Wyatt* v. *Portsmouth NHS Trust (No 3)* [2005] EWHC 693 (Fam), [2005] 2 FLR 480 (hereafter *Wyatt III*); *Re Wyatt (a child) (medical treatment: continuation of order)* [2005] EWCA Civ 1181, [2005] 1 WLR 3995 (CA) (hereafter *Wyatt IV*); *Re Wyatt* [2006] EWHC 319 (Fam), [2006] 2 FLR 111 (hereafter *Wyatt V*).

7 *R (on the application of Burke)* v. *General Medical Council* [2004] EWHC 1879 (Admin), [2005] QB 424 (hereafter *Burke I*); *R (on the application of Burke)* v. *General Medical Council* [2005] EWCA Civ 1003, [2006] QB 273 (CA) (hereafter *Burke II*).

8 *An NHS Trust* v. *MB* [2006] EWHC 507 (Fam), [2006] 2 FLR 319 (hereafter *MB*).

9 It is not within the scope of this study to include cases relating to assisted suicides such as the cases of Miss B or Diane Pretty.

10 *Wyatt I.*

11 *Wyatt II; Wyatt III; Wyatt V.*

12 *Wyatt IV.*

13 *Burke I.*

14 *Burke II.*

15 *Burke* v. *United Kingdom*, European Court of Human Rights, Application No. 19807/06.

16 The name of the baby, the parents, the health-care trust and the doctors involved were all kept anonymous.

17 Even where doctors do have disabilities, this fact alone does not make them expert at living with all disabilities.

18 This has been recognised by the GMC who published guidelines suggesting that all medical schools incorporate disability equality training into their curriculum (GMC 2003). Medical schools vary on their progress in this regard. Furthermore, such training will only assist our future doctors, not the doctors currently practising. Further continued professional development is required in this regard.

19 This was recognised by Mr Wolfe (the applicant's solicitor) in *Burke I*, para. 35.

20 Judges also do not respect the views of nurses as much as those of doctors. See the discussion of *MB* below.

21 Despite a move to evidence-based practice, there remains an element of doubt in all diagnoses.

22 *Re J* [1993] Fam 15 (CA).

23 *Burke I*, para. 30

24 Ibid., para. 24.

25 *Wyatt I.*

26 Referred to in the judgment as Dr S I (Consultant in Paediatric Intensive Care) and Dr S N (Consultant Paediatric Neurologist).

27 *MB*, para. 26: five consultants in paediatric intensive care, two consultant paediatric neurologists and one consultant paediatric anaesthetist.

28 Ibid., para. 26: four further doctors, two consulted by the trust, two by the parents.

29 Ibid., para. 29.

30 Ibid., para. 27.

31 Ibid., para. 30 (emphasis added).

32 Ibid., para. 16 (original emphasis).

33 Ibid., para. 16.

34 Ibid., para. 42 and again at para. 45.

35 *Frenchay Healthcare National Health Service Trust* v. *S* [1994] 1 WLR 601 (CA) p. 609 (original emphasis).

36 *Airedale NHS Trust* v. *Bland* [1993] AC 789 (HL); *Re J* [1993] Fam 15 (CA); *Re C* [1996] 2 FLR 43; *Re F* [1989] 2 FLR 376; *Re B* [1987] 2 All ER 206.

37 This is a similar point to that made by Montgomery in reference to *Re B* [1988] AC 199 (HL): see Montgomery (1989: 401).

38 *Wyatt I*, para. 16.

39 *Wyatt IV*, para. 33.

40 Advice from guardian in *Wyatt IV*, para. 46.

41 *Wyatt IV*, para. 117.

42 Ibid., para. 26.

43 Ibid.

44 The parents, the trust and the guardian.
45 *MB*, para. 59.
46 *Burke II*, para. 33.
47 Ibid., para. 24.
48 *Wyatt IV*, para 87.
49 *MB*, para. 58.
50 Ibid., para. 62.
51 However, it should be noted that this criticism could apply equally to carers, parents and even possibly patients considering themselves.
52 *MB*, para. 102.
53 *Re C (A minor) (Medical treatment)* [1998] Lloyd's Law Reports Medical 1. Here, devout Orthodox Jewish parents opposed doctors' wishes not to resuscitate C if she stopped breathing. Like MB, the baby had spinal muscular atrophy and, in the doctors' view, was in the process of dying. The court authorised the action supported by the doctors.
54 *Wyatt IV*, paras 20–1 and 119.
55 *Wyatt IV*, paras 86 and 117; *MB*, para. 54.
56 *MB*, para. 24.

Bibliography

Addington-Hall, J. and Kalra, L. (2001) 'Who Should Measure Quality of Life?', *British Medical Journal*, 322: 1417–20.
Altman, B. M. (2001) 'Disability Definitions, Models, Classification Schemes, and Applications', in G. Albrecht, K. Seelman and M. Bury (eds), *Handbook of Disability Studies*, Thousand Oaks, CA: Sage.
Andrews, K. (1996) 'Misdiagnosis of the Vegetative State: Retrospective Study in a Rehabilitation Unit', *British Medical Journal*, 313: 13–16.
Andrews, L. B. (2002) *Future Perfect: Confronting Decisions About Genetics*, New York: Columbia University Press.
Asch, A. (1988) 'Distracted by Disability', *Cambridge Quarterly of Healthcare Ethics*, 7: 77–87.
—— (2001) 'Disability, Bioethics, and Human Rights', in G. Albrecht, K. Seelman and M. Bury (eds), *Handbook of Disability Studies*, Thousand Oaks, CA: Sage.
British Council of Disabled People (2000) *The New Genetics and Disabled People*, London: BCODP.
Brownsword, R. (2006) 'An Introduction to Legal Research'. Available HTTP: < http://www.wellcome.ac.uk/assets/wtx030897.pdf > (accessed 2 January 2007).
Cella, D. F. (1992) 'Quality of Life: The Concept', *Journal of Palliative Care*, 8: 8–13.
Corker, M. and Shakespeare, T. (2002) 'Mapping the Terrain', in M. Corker and T. Shakespeare (eds), *Disability/Postmodernity: Embodying Disability Theory*, London: Continuum.
Department of Constitutional Affairs (2007) *Mental Capacity Act 2005 Code of Practice*, London: HMSO.
Derrida, J. (1978) *Writing and Difference*, Chicago, IL: University of Chicago Press.
Dworkin, R. W. (1993) *Life's Dominion*, London: HarperCollins.
Foster, C. (2005) 'Burke: A Tale of Unhappy Endings', *Journal of Philosophy and International Law* , 4: 293–300.
—— (2006a) 'Re MB: At the Edge of Life and at the Edge of the Law', *Family Law Journal*, 67: 8–9.

—— (2006b) 'Re MB: Always Look on the Bright Side of Life', *Healthcare Risk Report*, 12: 23–24.

Frisch, M. B. (1994) *Quality of Life Inventory*, Minneapolis, MN: National Computer Systems.

Gallagher, H. G. (1995) 'Can We Afford Disabled People?', Fourteenth Annual James C. Hemphill Lecture, Rehabilitation Institute of Chicago, 7 September.

General Medical Council (2003) *Tomorrow's Doctors: Recommendations for Undergraduate Medical Education*, London: GMC.

Gerhart, K. A., Koziol-McLain, J., Lowenstein, S. R. and Whiteneck, G. (1994) 'Quality of Life Following Spinal Cord Injury: Knowledge and Attitude of Emergency Care Providers', *Annals of Emergency Medicine*, 23: 807–12.

Goble, C. (2003) 'Controlling Life?', in J. Swain, S. French and S. Cameron (eds), *Controversial Issues in a Disabling Society*, Buckingham: Open University Press.

Holland, J. A. and Webb, J. S. (1996) *Learning Legal Rules*, 6th edn, Oxford: Oxford University Press.

Hughes, B. and Paterson, P. (1997) 'The Social Model of Disability and the Disappearing Body: Towards a Sociology of Impairment', *Disability and Society*, 12: 325–40.

Kennedy, I. (1988) 'Patients, Doctors and Human Rights', in I. Kennedy (ed.), *Treat Me Right: Essays in Medical Law and Ethics*, Oxford: Clarendon Press.

Montgomery, J. (1989) 'Rhetoric and "Welfare"', *Oxford Journal of Legal Studies*, 9: 395–402.

—— (2000) 'Health Care Law for a Multi-Faith Society', in J. Murphy (ed.), *Ethnic Minorities, Their Families and the Law*, Oxford: Hart Publishing.

Morris, J. (1991) *Pride Against Prejudice: Transforming Attitudes to Disability*, London: Women's Press.

Parens, E. and Asch, A. (eds) (2000) *Prenatal Testing and Disability Rights*, Washington DC: Georgetown University Press.

Reinders, H. S. (2000) *The Future of the Disabled in Liberal Society: An Ethical Analysis*, Notre Dame, IN: University of Notre Dame Press.

Rothwell, P. M., McDowell, Z., Wong, C. K. and Dorman, P. J. (1997) 'Doctors and Patients Don't Agree: Cross-sectional Study of Patients' and Doctors' Assessments of Disability in Multiple Sclerosis', *British Medical Journal*, 314: 1580–3.

Royal College of Paediatrics and Child Health (2004) *Withholding or Withdrawing Life Sustaining Treatment in Children: A Framework for Practice*, 2nd edn, London: RCPCH.

Saraga, E. (1998) *Embodying the Social: Constructions of Difference*, London and New York: Routledge.

Sehgal, A., Galbraith, A., Chesney, M., Schoenfeld, P., Charles, G. and Lo, B. (1992) 'How Strictly Do Dialysis Patients Want Their Advance Directives Followed?', *Journal of the American Medical Association*, 267: 59–63.

Shakespeare, T. (1998) 'Choice and Rights: Eugenics, Genetics and Disability Equality', *Disability and Society*, 13: 665–81.

—— (2006) *Disability Rights and Wrongs*, London and New York: Routledge.

Testa, M. A. and Nackley, J. F. (1994) 'Methods for Quality of Life Studies', *Annual Review of Public Health*, 59: 535–59.

Thomas, C. and Corker, M. (2002) 'A Journey Around the Social Model', in M. Corker and T. Shakespeare (eds), *Disability/Postmodernity: Embodying Disability Theory*, London: Continuum.

Tremain, S. (2002) 'On the Subject of Impairment', in M. Corker and T. Shakespeare (eds), *Disability/Postmodernity – Embodying Disability Theory*, London: Continuum.

Walter, J. and Shannon, T. (1990) *Quality of Life: The New Medical Dilemma*, Mahwah, NJ: Paulist Press.

Ward, L. (2002) 'Whose Right to Choose? The "New" Genetics, Prenatal Testing and People with Learning Difficulties', *Critical Public Health*, 12: 187–200.

Wasserman, D., Bickenbach, J. and Wachbroit, R. (eds) (2005) *Quality of Life and Human Difference: Genetic Testing, Health Care, and Disability*, Cambridge: Cambridge University Press.

12 Prenatal screening for Down syndrome

Why we shouldn't?

Berge Solberg

Introduction

At the turn of the century, several Western countries introduced prenatal screening for Down syndrome. Technology became widely and easily available, and the combination of ultrasound and then blood tests made it possible to screen the entire pregnant population. For the first time in history, there was a chance of detecting, and eventually aborting, most instances of Down syndrome, and at relatively low cost.

Some countries chose not to offer early screening during pregnancy, using value-based arguments, often claiming solidarity to weaker members in society. Yet, the same countries typically accepted abortion and prenatal diagnosis based on previously established maternal-age criteria.

This chapter investigates and discusses from a philosophical perspective whether there is a relevant difference between offering prenatal tests to high-risk groups as opposed to the entire pregnant population. Is this an ethical question, or a matter of more effective ways to introduce and use new medical technology? To screen or not to screen, that is the question.

Autonomy: a primary argument for screening

An illustrative case is the recent history of maternity care in Denmark, where the Danish National Health Service produced the report *Prenatal Diagnosis and Risk Assessment* (Sundhedsstyrelsen 2003) proposing a 'paradigmatic change in prenatal practice'. This report described the former paradigm as one centred on the prevention of disability, a mind-set said to have emerged from twentieth-century eugenic ideas. This report further suggests that prenatal diagnosis has been continuously contaminated by this way of thinking until fairly recently, ideas which should be abandoned and replaced by a new paradigm inspired by one prominent value in particular: autonomy. This would mean that the success criteria for prenatal screening would not be prevention of disability through a greater number of selective abortions, nor in economical expenditure brought about by a reduction of children born with impairments. The new sole criterion for success would be that pregnant women (and their partners) could exercise freedom of choice when it came to prenatal testing for Down syndrome.

Autonomy and screening apparently then belong together? If the primary justification for having a test is to increase freedom of choice and deciding future life
directions, then, in principle, anyone who could benefit from such tests should
have equal access to it. While the risk of having a baby with Down syndrome
apparently increases with the age of the mother, every pregnancy involves a certain degree of risk, and thus, screening for Down syndrome seems to represent a
fair distribution of both medical technology and information for individuals to
be able to make autonomous decisions. In Denmark, as well as in most countries
introducing screening for Down syndrome, the larger question about the relation
between autonomy and the presumed 'burden' of eventually having a child with
Down syndrome has not been a major consideration. Since prenatal diagnosis had
been offered to Danish women over the age of thirty-five years since the beginning of the 1980s, this debate appeared to have been settled. If one agrees with A,
one has to agree with B, the argument went. And in 2004, prenatal screening for
Down syndrome was introduced in Denmark.

At the same time, the expert group producing the report emphasised that
autonomy does not always mean 'a free choice from the uppermost shelf' (Sundhedsstyrelsen 2003). Autonomy and free choice are always defined within certain
limits, a claim few philosophers would protest. Relevant limits in this case concerned the choice of prenatal tests. Pregnant women were offered these tests based
on a certain risk assessment. They could choose whether they wanted to test for
Down syndrome or not, but not which tests they wanted. Interestingly, this leads
us to another argument for screening.

The not so hidden agenda: improving the accounts

Whether the world is changed by ideas or whether changes are caused by more
materialistic forces is a set of classical philosophical and political questions and
arguments. The reason why western countries put prenatal screening for Down
syndrome on the agenda has at least something to do with the development of
new technologies, most notably breakthroughs in ultrasound diagnosis in the
1990s. High-resolution pictures, improved interpretive skills, and the detection
of more 'soft markers' for disease and impairments enabled the way for ultrasound implementation early in pregnancy. The so-called 'thick neck-fold' has
been central in identifying Down syndrome (Nicolaides *et al.* 1992; Spencer
et al. 1999; Taipale *et al.* 1997), and an increased amount of fluid in the neck of
the foetus is also a possible sign of Down syndrome. Why this technology made
the 'autonomy paradigm' possible becomes more visible if contrasted with its
test-predecessor, amniocentesis.

Amniocentesis was and is an invasive technology. The needle enters the womb,
and such an intervention increases the risk of miscarriage. The risk is not dramatically high: about one out of a hundred pregnant women tested will abort as
a result of this pinprick. But the total number of losses would be unbearable for
health services worldwide if every pregnant woman were offered the possibility
of amniocentesis.

Denmark, along with Italy, has had the greatest reported use of amniocentesis in Europe, something which has been morally quite costly for Danish health services (Sundhedsstyrelsen 2003: 127). The number of foetuses without Down syndrome whose lives were lost as a consequence of amniocentesis was much higher than the number of foetuses detected with Down syndrome (Getz and Kirkengen 2003). By contrast, ultrasound in combination with blood tests could be offered to the entire pregnant population without having a negative impact on the balance of results: more foetuses with Down syndrome could then be detected while fewer foetuses without Down syndrome would be lost (Sundhedsstyrelsen 2003).

The point I am making here is that Denmark and other countries offering early ultrasound screening did not introduce it in order to rid themselves of people with Down syndrome. The new technological solution had its own internal logic: more (and even most) cases of Down syndrome could be detected, and at a lower cost of human life. No matter how one chooses to view this, either from an economic or human perspective, the balance was better than it had been.

Of course, this might be good news if plans were intended to reduce the number of future people with Down syndrome. But based on the lesson learnt from Danish eugenic history (and other countries), such intentions were increasingly discredited. More and more, the dominant values concerning prenatal diagnosis in most western societies today are those of free choice and self-determination, and the new technological possibilities suit these ideals very well. After all, the more risk-free tests available, the more choices are made available. Giving everyone the choice of having (or not) a baby with Down syndrome by offering non-invasive tests increases the autonomy of pregnant women and/or their partners, no matter what choice they make. To test or not to test, carrying an affected foetus to term or aborting, became solely all about autonomy! For the Danish National Health service, this seemed to be a win-win situation: the transition from invasive to non-invasive technology combined with the expansion of free choice seemed to represent some sort of ethical progress.

Arguments against screening

Scrutinising technology sheds light on how the screening debate is contextualised in different ways. For instance, Denmark's neighbour country Norway has had stricter maternal age criteria than Denmark (thirty-eight years old), and as a consequence, the number of amniocentesis procedures performed in Norway and the number of unwanted losses has been fewer. If Norway were to introduce prenatal early screening for Down syndrome, the total number of amniocentesis procedures might increase dramatically and so too the number of unintentionally lost healthy foetuses. The 'internal logic' of the technology then, did not clear the way for autonomous choice. In practice this meant that the 'push' from the techno-medical establishment towards screening was not as great as it would have been if it had represented a clear step forward when compared to previous patterns.

In fact, resistance towards introducing early ultrasound screening was quite high in Norway, even though the Norwegian National Health Service offered testing for Down syndrome for women in the 'high risk' category. One example of this resistance is that the Norwegian Minister of Health recommended in 1999 that a leading Norwegian ultrasound specialist stop a planned study on early ultrasound (NTB 1999), fearing that the study would encourage early ultrasound screening.

A central argument against screening in Norway and elsewhere is a version of an expressivist argument. The expressivist argument is articulated, among others, by Adrienne Asch's 'any–particular distinction' (Asch 2000): to abort a foetus when the pregnancy is unwanted is to abort 'any kind' of foetus, whereas to abort a foetus with (for instance) Down syndrome is to abort a 'particular one' with characteristics that are shared by other members of society. While an abortion can belong to the private sphere, concerning primarily the woman and the foetus in her womb, a selective abortion affects other people or groups of people in society and is then a public and societal matter. This is the ethical-political dimension of selective abortions, according to Asch. In a selective abortion, certain ideas about the anticipated quality of life (or absence thereof), about burdens or happiness (or not), and about the meaning of family life provide premises for making the decision. This line of thinking leads to a conclusion that selective abortions express discriminatory or offensive attitudes to (particular groups of) disabled people.

Nancy Press (2000) argues not to focus on the message from a specific abortion or on the woman having an abortion, but rather on the meaning of the offered possibility of prenatal testing itself. Her point fits well with the public debate in Norway, and opens up a possible ethical distinction between a high-risk strategy and screening. The offer of testing to a small high-risk group has different implications than the offer of testing to a larger number of low-risk pregnant women. In the case of the former, prenatal tests can be legitimated on the grounds of a conscious knowledge and anxiety about one's own 'natural' risk. In the case of the latter, the message from a National Health Service would seem to be much clearer: Down syndrome is such a potentially severe threat to a 'good family life', that abortion might be a better solution, at least for some.

The expressivist argument has a strong standing in Norwegian public debates, occurring in various versions. One creative version was presented in the spring of 2007 on national Norwegian television, when Marthe Goksøyr presented her own video diary (NRK 2007). Marthe has Down syndrome and filmed herself entering the laboratory of a medical genetics department with her video camera, asking the staff there why parents wanted to terminate people 'like her'. The result (an extremely uncomfortable situation for the geneticists) did not in itself constitute proof that the expressivist argument is correct, but the uncomfortable situation needs to be understood and explained.

A credible response from the geneticists might have been one provided by several bio-ethicists: terminating a foetus is not terminating Marthe or someone else, but rather only about terminating a foetus. This position is argued by several well-known bioethicists, among them John Harris (1998) and Peter Singer (1994). Tom Shakespeare formulated such a position as follows: 'it seems intuitively true that if it is permissible to terminate pregnancy at all, it is permissible to terminate in the case of disability' (Shakespeare 2006: 93). One perhaps tends to forget that we are thinking and talking about foetuses here, and that many of us would find it permissible to terminate a pregnancy even when it does *not* involve a potential disease or impairment.

But such a response does not seem to consider all of the messages regarding the central question of this chapter, that of screening: some messages and signals are more intense than others. Perhaps it is not the permissibility of terminating that is necessarily at issue but rather the permissibility of actively arranging situations where terminating is one of the endpoints? Such a step goes too far judgementally for the (family) lives of people with Down syndrome, according to critics. But is this critique a sustainable one?

The struggle for recognition

Many people with Down syndrome and their families feel that the message from prenatal screening hurts, diminishes and devalues them in various ways. One mother quite well known in Norway who has a child with Down syndrome for-mulated it this way in the media: 'We find that health professionals talk about people with Down syndrome as if they were defect cars that shouldn't have been on the market' (Borud 2000).

If this were a representative experience for disabled people and their rela-tives, it would be easy to conclude that prenatal screening is at least *perceived* as offensive. But isn't reality more complex? Disabled people and their families do not always experience a sense of diminishment when confronted with prenatal screening and diagnosis. Perhaps the variable here is not primarily one of ideas or values, but rather which impairment is being considered? After all, the conditions of spina bifida and cystic fibrosis have not led to the same degree of controversy and intensity in public bioethical debates as has Down syndrome. A simple but convincing way to establish this claim is that a recent search in the Retriever archive for Norwegian media provided 513 hits for the combined terms 'Down syndrome' and 'prenatal diagnosis', whereas a search for 'spina bifida' and 'pre-natal diagnosis' resulted in twenty-four hits, and 'cystic fibrosis' and 'prenatal diagnosis' in only fifteen hits (A-tekst 2008). One reason for this might be that the overall incidence of Down syndrome is higher than the incidence of spina bifida and cystic fibrosis. But this may not be the main reason. The main reason, in my opinion, has something to do with the fact that some impairments and disabilities constitute what Stainton (2003) has called 'strong identity characteristics', and this then makes the expressivist critique more relevant when considering Down syndrome compared to other impairments.

Stainton's point is that prenatal screening for intellectual disabilities can in itself be viewed as an expression of an identity-based oppression. The fact that people with intellectual disabilities neither objectively suffer, nor experience any more or less sadness or joy than the rest of us seems to count for little, even among those who are otherwise concerned with the implications of testing and elimi-nation for other types of disabilities, according to Stainton (2003: 538). In his view, then, prenatal screening for Down syndrome may not only have potentially negative consequences for people with Down syndrome and for their families. We could instead turn it around: prenatal screening for intellectual disabilities may be an indication that something has gone wrong in society with regards to identity construction. And Stainton suspects that the origin of the problem is in the history of modernity, where the intellect is so highly valued.

I believe Stainton is correct, at least in his focus on identity. Down syndrome is different from spina bifida, well illustrated in Norway where a former Minister of Environmental Protection, Guro Fjellanger, had spina bifida, while no one with Down syndrome is likely to become a minister. Fjellanger was dependent on crutches and wheelchairs and accessible settings in order to do her job. Having Down syndrome is not an impairment that can be compensated for so easily, at least not to the extent that one could perform most duties of a governmental minister. A person with Down syndrome would not just be different, but *too different* to include in politics at that level.

Some people might then draw the conclusion that prenatal screening for, and the abortion of, foetuses with spina bifida is morally more problematic than Down syndrome, because the latter is potentially a much more severe condition than the former. The former is not necessarily even a hindrance to becoming a minister. But this logic fails to explain public controversies about Down syndrome and the lack of public controversies about spina bifida. The point is rather that prenatal screening for Down syndrome highlights the problematic nature of intellectual impairments in our societies. People with Down syndrome and their families face what Charles Taylor (1995) has called a 'struggle for recognition' to a larger extent than people with spina bifida and their families.

Terminating foetuses, terminating burdens or terminating identities?

John Harris (1998: 215) has subjected such expressivist relations to critique in his 'argument from Beethoven'. Beethoven, it will be recalled, was deaf. But to abort a foetus with 'Beethoven syndrome' is not to abort Beethoven, but rather as Harris contends, it is just to abort a foetus. Harris's argument can be clarified thus: everyone would prefer to have babies with two legs instead of one leg. If we could prevent having a one-legged baby by postponing conception by one month, we would and should postpone conception. To then claim that our actions were offensive to people with only one leg, or that we were expressing oppressive identity characteristics, would be absurd. So in Harris' view, regarding debates on disability, respect and recognition are non-starters: it is 'better' to have children without Down syndrome in the same way that it is better to have children with two legs instead of one. According to Harris, that is what prenatal diagnosis is all about.

Harris presupposes that a foetus is not a moral person: it is, then, 'a nothing'. And thus, preventing impaired children by abortion or postponed conception amounts to one and the same thing. This position is of course valid if you happen to believe that an embryo or a foetus has no moral value whatsoever. But since this position represents only one possible interpretation of the moral standing of the foetus, and one that is marginal in most western cultures, it is a position that does not adequately provide meaning to the widespread feeling that prenatal diagnosis and selective abortion are related in important ways to the politics of disability.

An alternative point of departure would be that most people think we should ascribe some moral value to the foetus. Even where women can have abortion on demand, without having to justify their decision, there is still a tacit requirement for a kind of 'private' justification. To abort because the pregnancy collides with an unexpected holiday in the Greek islands is not sufficient justification in the minds of most people. The (presumed) burden does not outweigh the kind of moral value that is typically assigned to the foetus. This vague notion of morality strongly suggests that preventing disability by abortion has a 'moral cost'. I am not claiming that the moral cost is the killing of a person, but simply preserving the common intuition that some moral cost is involved.

In contrast, if future people with Down syndrome could be prevented by postponing certain conceptions or taking a pill before conception, there would be no moral cost involved in such prevention, because abortion is excluded from the options. The expression of such prevention is that forthcoming parents want children without Down syndrome. But everyone knows that forthcoming parents as a basis want children without disease and impairments. The message to be inferred from prenatal screening, on the other hand, is that (family) life with Down syndrome is so negatively valued that the morally problematic action of abortion could be preferable.

Since opinions differ as to what extent any abortion is morally problematic, this means that the grade of offensiveness also has to differ. I call this the 'gradualist view of offensiveness'. This means among other things that it is logically impossible to defend a position where one denies any kind of moral value to the foetus, while simultaneously claiming that prenatal screening is offensive. Here, Harris is quite correct. A provoked abortion must be viewed as an event that involves a 'moral cost' if one is to claim that there is a message sent from prenatal screening programs and selective abortions to disabled people in society. And in most cases, this would be viewed as having a moral cost.

On the other hand, a gradualist view of offensiveness is not just dependent on the moral judgement of abortion. It is a necessary but not sufficient condition. In addition, it is dependent, as stated earlier in this chapter, on the nature of the disease or disability in question. When Norwegian women still chose selective abortion on the basis of spina bifida, after Guro Fjellanger became a national Minister and a public figure, they were not 'terminating the minister'. They still knew there might be potentially substantial burdens connected to (family) life with a child with spina bifida, and that the spectrum of the impairment could vary dramatically. So, most of them opted for termination.[1]

To abort a foetus with Down syndrome, on the other hand, is probably to a certain extent *to abort the person that is too different to become a minister.* Down syndrome has a stronger identity characteristic than spina bifida. When the majority culture is able to become acquainted with a person with spina bifida as a minister, or a university student, an artist or a gay person, the same majority culture will in all probability and in most cases still 'know' a person with Down syndrome as a person with Down syndrome. The task of getting beyond the impairment will be much larger. Of course one could argue that there are often significant burdens related to having a child with Down syndrome (and the burdens will not disappear when the child grows up). But to a larger degree, it is the identity that is terminated in a prenatal screening for Down syndrome, and not first and foremost the future burden. The difference, and not the anticipated or potential burden, is at stake. One proof of that is the shock women get when they unknowingly give birth to a child with Down syndrome. Getting a postnatal Down syndrome diagnosis, the parents feel shocked, angry, devastated, overwhelmed, depressed, stunned and helpless (Skotko 2005). This shock is probably not primarily caused by the thoughts on the burdens lying ahead but rather provoked by the *difference* between the wanted child and the real child.

The strong identity-forming character of Down syndrome is based partly on the fact that people with the syndrome typically have intellectual/cognitive impairments and partly on the fact that this impairment is at the same time thought to mean a happy life for the person with Down syndrome, such as a cheerful way of being. Additionally, a person with Down syndrome is recognisable on the street because of her or his facial characteristics. All of these factors add up to Down syndrome being constructed as 'pure difference' in societies such as Norway. Whereas Fragile X syndrome is understood as a disease, for instance, and is understood to belong to the 'domain' of medical geneticists and genetic counsellors, Down syndrome is a symbol for a different way of 'being human' in the public sphere: a way that is vulnerable but also one valuable and worth protecting.

If this argument is correct, people with Down syndrome and their families have good reasons to be offended by prenatal screening offers. It is a basic need to feel that you live in a society where you and your child are welcome. It seems then that the expressivist position has something relevant to contribute, especially with regards to the larger implications of intellectual impairments such as Down syndrome. Under attack here are the identities and descriptions that people with Down syndrome can create and thrive with. The greater the human and economic costs, coupled with societally sanctioned prenatal tests and service-supports designed to give parents the choice of preventing babies with Down syndrome, the more difficult it becomes for people with Down syndrome to have the positive aspects of their identity recognised by society.

At the same time, there is a paradox here: precisely because Down syndrome has been successfully constructed as a 'difference' in the Norwegian public sphere, the termination of foetuses with trisomy 21 has become problematic. Framing impairment in order to make it a question of identity may be an empowering strategy in many arenas in society, whereas in prenatal diagnostics it leads to confrontation and a feeling among some people that the practice is offensive. As Lynn Gillam has remarked, to have someone look at your life from the outside, making judgements about how fulfilling and happy you are – or not – must be deeply offensive. But at the same time Gillam warns against equating this feeling of offence with discrimination. She writes, 'The fact selective abortion is offensive to many people with disabilities does not in itself make selective abortion discriminatory to those who are offended by it' (Gillam 1999: 170).

'Offence' is a rather vague kind of harm, and there are other powerful ethical considerations that deserve consideration. If critical voices have been thoroughly heard in a country such as Norway, could it be that the Danish voices for autonomy and maternal care have been ignored? If it is a fact that intelligence is valued in modern societies, and if we recognise that, then shouldn't autonomy and not just a discussion on 'burdens' be relevant?

Autonomy as trump

Returning to my claim, perhaps the paradigm shift in Denmark was mainly motivated by the efficiency of new technology and not by considerations of autonomy. But even if this claim is correct, it does not make the issue of autonomy irrelevant or invalid. Perhaps quite the opposite: references to the value of autonomy provide a very common and powerful response to new technological possibilities.

There are several important reasons why autonomy should play a central role in medical genetics. Many western countries, and indeed the Scandinavian countries, have histories of eugenic practice, where violation of autonomy and a lack of respect for individual preferences and choices were at the core of mistakes in medical genetics (Broberg and Roll-Hansen 1996). Autonomous choice seems to be a bulwark against oppression. Autonomy and self-determination also seem to represent a highly relevant perspective in choices that will affect individuals dramatically. If we are allowed to choose between different toothpastes, there seems to be little sense in restricting individual choice in more important matters. The logic should instead be the other way around: autonomy and self-determining freedom are primarily important when there is something very significant at stake.

What is seen as offensive about prenatal screening for Down syndrome is precisely the same factors that make autonomy and choice extremely relevant to this practice. Down syndrome represents not a disease, but rather a radical difference. This difference challenges the idea and the purpose of reproduction. No one denies that having a baby with Down syndrome is a shock, although it is known that most parents eventually adapt to the situation. It is a potentially greater challenge to become reconciled to the fact that your foetus has Down syndrome, than to become reconciled to the fact of an unwanted pregnancy. But it is only in the last instance that autonomy and choice become 'obvious' relevant factors in, for example, a country such as Norway. Having a seriously impaired child provides major and long-term challenges to parents. It seems odd to deny, then, that autonomous choice is a matter of concern in such instances when it is a matter of course that an unplanned child will have a serious and similarly long-term impact.

There is increasing evidence for the argument that Down syndrome is not a threat to a good family life. Many myths exist about such family lives, a prominent one being that the parents of disabled children divorce more often than other parents. In fact, the opposite is true (Lundeby and Tøssebro 2007). One might further argue that people who believe that a family member with impairments is not conducive to a good (family) life do not know what they are talking about. But the problem is that exactly the same argument can be used against autonomy and choice with regards to an unplanned child. Yet, it is not the case that one tries to convince women about to undergo abortions that a life with an unplanned child would in fact be productive and fulfilling. One accepts her/their autonomous choice, partly because these questions may have more than one answer, and partly because we believe that the person whose life and body are most centrally affected has the right to come up with the answers and choices that feel right for her.

Prenatal screening for Down syndrome provides all pregnant women with equal rights and alternatives. It represents the fair distribution of technology and information – and such universal access in Denmark prevents unequal treatment based on resources, education, age or place of residence. In Norway, in 2007, pregnant women who had higher education and were under the age of thirty-eight knew that if they told their doctor that they suffered from severe anxiety during pregnancy, they would be referred for an early ultrasound check. If this were not the case, a woman would ordinarily be offered ultrasound only in the second trimester, which is a poorer predictor of Down syndrome. If we consider the neckfold scan and the blood test as social goods, there seems to be a fairer distribution of these goods in Denmark than in Norway.

Shifting the focus from *offence* to *autonomy*, it seems as if the Danish prenatal screening programme reflects and enhances important values in western cultures. The possibility that people with Down syndrome and/or their families might be offended to some degree must be weighed against the harm done by suppressing pregnant women's freedom to exercise choice, as Edwards (2004) has argued. Since the feeling of being offended is a rather vague one, and since it is unlikely to result in concrete and harmful consequences such as a worsening of attitudes towards disabled people or a reduction in the standards of care, as Shakespeare has pointed out (Shakespeare 2006: 96), autonomy does seem to be the more important consideration. Offering early ultrasound and medical genetic services seems to enhance the autonomy of every pregnant woman and also improves the quality of their pregnancies. Each year in Denmark, about 60,000 pregnant women will enjoy a pregnancy that involves less anxiety and allows them increased control over their future lives. The chance of a small number of families with Down syndrome taking offence, and possibility of criticism from disability movements, cannot be decisive, if we accept this version of priorities as the correct one. Following this line of reasoning, it seems that we have arrived at a position whereby the expressivist critique of prenatal diagnosis is acknowledged as relevant but outweighed by the argument that to suppress the autonomy of pregnant women would be far more harmful.

However, could it be that the case for autonomy is too simple and superficial? Do we really know that prenatal screening for Down syndrome increases the autonomy of pregnant women or leads to reduced levels of anxiety and an increased quality of pregnancy? Since our apparent conclusion rests substantially on the autonomy-argument, we need to investigate the empirical basis for this argument before arriving at more certain judgements.

Ethics and screening: about pregnancy rather than disability?

There are certain challenges related to all sorts of screening projects. In the end these challenges can be summed up under the category of 'information'. But what gives rise to this information problem is closely connected to the phenomena of false positive and false negative screening results. Screening is often compared to fishing with a net. If the mesh is too wide, some of the fish you want to catch will escape. If the mesh is too narrow, fewer of the fish you want will escape, but more unwanted fish will be caught. So there needs to be a compromise of some kind.

In prenatal screening for Down syndrome the 'unwanted fishes' are the healthy babies that are unnecessarily assigned a risk label, where the neck-fold scan and blood tests lead to the mothers of these babies being identified as belonging to a high-risk group. But they are 'false positive', in the sense that amniocentesis would reveal that their foetuses did not have Down syndrome.[2] Continuing with the fish-net metaphor, there are other 'fish' representing another problem: the neck-fold scan will not be able to detect all foetuses with Down syndrome. About 10–15 per cent will not be discovered, in spite of this test, thus representing the 'wanted fish that pass through the net', those that test 'false negative'.

False positives and false negatives generate at least three separate medical-ethical problems. When screening the entire Danish pregnant population of nearly 60,000 women, about 3,000 of them will be 'unnecessarily' worried, according to estimates from the Ministry of Health (Sundhedsstyrelsen 2003). So, the first problem is the one of unnecessary anxiety and a spoiled quality of pregnancy. Second, about thirty of these women will lose their 'normal' baby at a later stage as a result of amniocentesis procedures used only to establish that the positive 'diagnosis' was false; this second problem is the more well-recognised one of unwanted loss brought about by invasive diagnostics. Third, between ten and fifteen women will still give birth to a child with Down syndrome, even though they go through all the scans and blood tests; the third problem is the one of getting exactly the 'sort' of baby you thought you had decided not to get.

What is the relation between these three clinical-ethical challenges and autonomy? Well, suddenly 'autonomy' becomes a field of empirical investigation. Without going deeply into the philosophical debates on the meaning of autonomy, it seems reasonable to assert that autonomous choices have something to do with informed and free choices. A lack of information or lack of understanding of the purpose of a medical test does not foster autonomy. Similarly, a choice made on the basis of irrational anxiety and fear is not what we usually think of as the celebrated 'autonomous choice'.

There is a small but rapidly growing body of empirical research on this subject. A 2006 study by Müller *et al.* concluded that nuchal translucency (NT) screening (early ultrasound scan) for Down syndrome does not increase anxiety or depression levels in pregnancy. In fact, the study showed that women who underwent screening were less likely to be anxious compared with those who were not offered screening (Müller *et al.* 2006). This finding so enthused the ethicists Chervenak *et al.* that they felt compelled to state the following: 'We have argued that routine obstetric ultrasound is an important autonomy-enhancing strategy ... This is further evidence that first-trimester risk assessment enhances the autonomy of pregnant women without biopsychosocial harm' (Chervenak *et al.* 2006: 355).

But 'empirical evidence' points in different directions. One study that Müller *et al.* use to support their findings is a 2003 Swedish study which concluded that early ultrasound screening does not cause more anxiety or concerns about the health of the baby than a routine scan later in pregnancy does. But the authors are nevertheless in doubt as to whether their conclusions are fully reliable. They observed that levels of anxiety among respondents in the control group were significantly higher than levels presented in other studies, including another study performed in Sweden at the same time. The authors suggest that information about the aim of the study with a strong focus on foetal abnormality may have made all the women more aware of the possibility that something may go wrong (Öhman *et al.* 2004). These elements of doubt led the authors to carry out a new study some years later using a qualitative design which focused on women's reactions to a false positive test, with a conclusion that totally contradicts that of Müller: 'A false positive test of foetal screening for Down syndrome by ultrasound examination may cause strong reactions of anxiety and even rejection of pregnancy. The prevalence of such reactions and possible long term effects need further investigation' (Öhman *et al.* 2006: 64).

A 2007 study of the Danish screening programme found that the pregnant women's motives for having an NT-scan were based on rationales that hindered an informed choice being made (Lou *et al.* 2007). The most important motives for wanting an NT-scan were to do with reassurance, choice, expectations about the scan being a happy event and, last but not least, on the idea that the test was right because of its approval by the Danish health-care system.

Put more simply, the Danish study showed that a typical behavioural pattern for pregnant women is to have an NT-scan in order to ensure that their child does not have Down syndrome. Most of the women are fairly certain about this before they come for the scan, and this contributes to the perception that the scan is a happy event for the mother and the father. From the perspective of Chervenak *et al.*, these factors would not argue against the rationale of enhanced autonomy. Having the possibility of an early ultrasound in order to get in touch with the foetus at an earlier stage through the medium of screen and sharing a positive experience with one's future child can be seen as an expression of increased autonomy.

Although such an understanding of autonomy might be in line with the thinking of Chervenak *et al.*, it is definitely not in line with the view of the medical establishment, as evidenced by the strong reaction of the European Committee for Medical Ultrasound Safety (ECMUS) among others to 'souvenir scanning'. In 2006, they stated that ultrasound scans should not be performed solely for the production of souvenir images or for the recording of a foetus or embryo, arguing that, 'Very little information is available regarding possible subtle biological effects of diagnostic levels of ultrasound on the developing human embryo or fetus, and the possibility of developmental effects in the brain cannot be ruled out' (ECMUS 2006).

Of course from a medical point of view, an NT-scan has a diagnostic benefit because it can assess the risk of Down syndrome, and getting an early scan in order to have this information increases the autonomy of the individual. But if Danish women are primarily interested in prenatal screening because they want to experience a happy event, are they choosing the scan for the 'wrong' reason? The only acceptable motivation from a medical perspective is that women take the scan because they want to rule out the possibility of having a baby with Down syndrome and are prepared to take the 'rational' consequences of that risk estimate. So again, the 'autonomous choice' can be questioned according to whether it is (actually) informed, rational and free.

Feminist perspectives also question the idea that the greater the range of medical-technological choices, the greater the autonomy one has. The supposition is that women want tests and technological assistance in order to be better informed and more in control. But at the same time, the battery of tests and scans performed can only be interpreted by experts. The ultrasound machine devalues the former perception of risk, that of high maternal age, and a woman's own opinion about the due date (Saetnan 2000). Only ultrasound can provide a correct answer to these questions. But not every pregnant woman is capable of understanding this technology in order to interpret the status of the foetus. The ultrasound pictures 'lies' in many ways, and what you see is not necessarily what you get, in the sense that one cannot really understand these images without years of advanced training. So, as this line of critique goes, women again become dependent on medical experts (mainly men) who can interpret the advanced technological results, and tell them what is going on in their own pregnancies, including what they should fear or not.

From a philosophical view, the link between choice(s) and freedom is questionable. We know that in some areas of life, more choices do not generate more freedom or autonomy. In some instances, it is in fact the opposite, with marriage being a highly illustrative example. The quality of a marriage is not increased by introducing new and freely chosen partners every day. If you believe in marriage, you believe that the practice has value precisely because it does not permit choices of this type. The same type of argumentation could be applied to parenthood. As Simo Vehmas has pointed out, parenthood is essentially an unconditional project (2002). You do not become a more autonomous or freer parent by being given the choice of throwing away your children when you become tired of them. Again, it is the opposite: good parenthood is good precisely because it is unconditional.

However, this last point raises the question of when one becomes a parent in relation to prenatal diagnosis. It is not necessary to open that discussion here but rather to make the point that there is no inevitable link between introducing the choice of neck-fold screening in pregnancy and that of enhancing autonomy.

The link can be questioned from several empirical and normative perspectives. Indeed, two other ethical challenges that follow from screening strengthen this conclusion. Hall *et al.* concluded in 2000 that 'a false negative result on prenatal screening seems to have a small adverse effect on parental adjustment, evident two to six years after the birth of an affected child' (Hall *et al.* 2000: 407). In Denmark this has already lead to wrongful-birth trials brought against the National Health Service (Skovmand 2005). And the potential harm of losing a perfectly healthy and wanted baby as a result of prenatal screening (and subsequent amniocentesis) that 'everybody else' utilises has not been empirically investigated yet.

All these aspects are specific to prenatal screening for Down syndrome but do not apply to the same degree for a high-risk strategy where maternal age is the reason for offering such medical genetic services. The main reason for this is that older pregnant women probably have a more conscious understanding of their risk. Being forty years old and pregnant, there is a substantial increased risk in pregnancy. Prenatal diagnosis can be perceived as the 'treatment' of an anxiety related to this risk, and not as society's view on people with Down syndrome. Older pregnant women are fewer in number and can receive better counselling. Their choices might be better informed. Informed consent might be reachable.

To screen or not to screen?

What is challenging about prenatal screening is the ethical complexity of the phenomenon. Principal and empirical questions arise, and it is difficult to follow all the separate and sometimes interwoven threads, and still be able to take a general and balanced view. What follows is an attempt at summing up the sides of the argument, and moving towards a potential conclusion.

I have identified two major strands of ethical thinking in relation to prenatal screening for Down syndrome. The first can be labelled the *disability discussion:* my main focus in describing it has been on the impact from screening on the struggle for recognition by people with intellectual impairments and their families, the potential for screening to cause offence, and the relevance of the expressivist critique. The primary pro-argument for prenatal screening in the disability discussion is to give pregnant women the choice of not becoming mothers to impaired/disabled children. Screening, so the argument goes, allows more women not to have a radically different child or a child that will prevent a good family life or otherwise constitute a burden.

The second discussion can be labelled the *good-maternal-care discussion.* Since only a very small minority of pregnant women carry a baby with Down syndrome, and prenatal screening includes everyone, we cannot limit the focus only to those few. Prenatal screening changes how pregnancy and being pregnant are understood and experienced. My main focus here has been on the adverse consequences followed by false alarms and false negatives but also on the information and understanding of the entire pregnant population. The primary pro-argument for Down syndrome-screening in this discourse, on the other hand, is the fact that the test is free of risk, hence the restrictions connected to amniocentesis did not come into play and more women could benefit from a reduction of anxiety early in pregnancy.

These two discussions remain for the most part separate and discussed in different journals. Philosophers, bioethicists and disability theorists tend to favour the first discussion. The principal ethical questions seem to lie there. In medical journals and in clinical ethics, one finds more of the second discussion. There is a long tradition in medicine for defining 'good treatment' of a patient as a matter of balancing risk against benefit. As long as the pregnant woman can be presented as the patient, and the more controversial topic of the foetus as the real patient is disregarded, this discussion is fruitful and functional.

Both discussions deserve the name 'ethical discussions'. But what happens if we try to bring them together? Will it provide any guidance on the question of whether we should screen or not screen? An interesting effect of attempting to join the two perspectives is that the critical potential in each perspective is strengthened by the other. From a critical disability perspective, abortion is a problematic way of preventing the birth of a disabled child. But if the national health service provide a screening service that results in massive false-alarm problems, tragically false negative-problems, huge economical expenditures and selective abortions based on inaccurate information, the costs (in the extended meaning of the word) to a society which accepts the necessity of preventing a disabled child increase dramatically. This means a further devaluing of the disease or impairment/disability in question, in terms of 'worth-living' dimensions. The implication seems to be that these costs are acceptable, because it is vital that every pregnant woman has the opportunity to terminate a foetus with Down syndrome. Put in a utilitarian framework: Since the 'costs' of a prenatal screening program are substantial, and costs need to be justified, the burden of Down syndrome and the harm of getting a baby with Down syndrome have to increase. Only the possible prevention of great harm can outweigh the human and economical costs of the screening programme. The expressivist critique appears more relevant to a screening programme for Downs syndrome compared to a high-risk strategy.

Similarly, the critical potential in the good-maternal-care perspective is strengthened by bringing in the disability perspective. If we could agree that impairment is a part of life and not necessarily a tragic one, then pregnant women should experience less anxiety and the need for a battery of risk-estimating tests would be reduced. Medical technology would play a less central role in pregnancy, while the pregnant woman would still be in charge and could more easily indulge in this part of life.

The point of this chapter is not that prenatal testing for Down syndrome is unethical: it is rather that the supporters of early screening in the whole pregnant population for Down syndrome have had an all too easy time of it so far. Very seldom are they confronted with the combined critical perspectives of both the disability discussion and the good-maternal-care discussion. The combined critique suggests that early screening for Down syndrome may cause more harm than good. And the critique claims that there is an ethical relevant difference between a high-risk strategy and population-based early screening.

There exists a third way out of the dilemma of early screening for Down syndrome. This third way would be to implement early screening because of its medical benefit for the foetus. The 'neck-fold' which is a marker for Down syndrome, is also a marker for different sorts of anomalies that are associated with kinds of heart failure, among others, that may be treatable (Hyett *et al.* 1997). With a legitimate therapeutic focus, controversial aspects such as selection and negative attitudes to disabled people are downplayed. Even the opposite could be the case, since many malformations that would have led to an abortion decision earlier can now be treated and the babies would be carried to term. At the same time, therapeutic legitimating is more in line with the good-maternal-care perspective: mothers are not offered a test in order to find out whether the foetus is an enemy or a friend, but rather because it could be beneficial for the foetus.

Today, the medical challenge is to be able to prove the therapeutic benefit(s) from early screening. The benefits have to be significant should they override the combined critical perspective. Until such benefits are proven (if they ever will be), to screen or not to screen is a powerful ethical question involving deep identity questions with regards to impairment/disability, pregnancy and technology.

Notes

1 An additional motive for terminating a foetus with spina bifida is the risk of getting a child with an intellectual disability. But this motive is not directly dependent on how the identity of people with spina bifida is constructed in public. Intellectual disability is not an issue when it comes to well-situated people with spina bifida in Norwegian public life.

2 The term 'false positive' has generated controversies and misunderstandings in this debate because it easily leads one to conclude that a pregnant woman receives the diagnosis Down syndrome, and then this turns out to be false. If the amniocentesis test was positive, the mother had an abortion and it turned out that the aborted foetus did not have Down syndrome, this would then have been a false positive. But this happens extremely seldom, if at all. What we are talking about in ultrasound screening is getting a risk label. Risk is about statistics, and in that sense 'high risk' can be true even if the baby in the end is perfectly healthy. So it might be true that the term 'false positive' could be misleading, and because of that, the alternative term 'false alarm' has been proposed as preferable.

Bibliography

Asch, A. (2000) 'Why I Haven't Changed My Mind on Prenatal Diagnosis', in E. Parens and A. Asch (eds), *Prenatal Testing and Disability Rights*, Washington, DC: Georgetown University Press.

A-tekst (2008) The digital retriever media-archive. Available at < http://www.retriever-info.com/atekst.php > (accessed 28 January 2008).

Borud, H. (2000) 'Vis respekt for våre barn' ('Show Respect for our Children'), Oslo: *Aftenposten*, 5 June.

Broberg, G. and Roll-Hansen, N. (1996) *Eugenics and the Welfare State: Sterilisation Policy in Denmark, Sweden, Norway and Finland*, Ann Arbor, MI: Michigan University Press.

Chervenak, F. A., McCullough, L. B and Chasen, S. T. (2006) 'Further Evidence for First-Trimester Risk Assessment As an Autonomy-Enhancing Strategy', *Ultrasound in Obstetrics and Gynecology*, 27: 355.

ECMUS (European Committee for Medical Ultrasound Safety) (2006), Available HTTP: < http://www.efsumb.org/efsumb/committees/Safety_Committee/Safety_Eng/2006%20 souvenir%20scanning%20statement.pdf > (accessed 3 January 2006).

Edwards, S. D. (2004) 'Disability, Identity and the "Expressivist Objection"', *Journal of Medical Ethics*, 30: 418–20.

Getz, L. and Kirkengen, A. L. (2003) 'Ultrasound Screening of Pregnancy: Advancing Technology, Soft Markers of Fetal Anomaly and Unacknowledged Ethical Dilemmas', *Social Science and Medicine*, 56: 2045–57.

Gillam, L. (1999) 'Prenatal Diagnosis and Discrimination Against the Disabled', *Journal of Medical Ethics*, 25: 163–71.

Harris, J. (1998) *Clones, Genes and Immortality*, Oxford: Oxford University Press.

Hyett, J. A., Perdu, M., Sharland, G. K., Fetal Cardiology Unit, Guy's Hospital, London, UK, Snijders, R. S. M. and Nicolaides, K. H. (1997) 'Increased Nuchal Translucency at 10–14 Weeks of Gestation As a Marker for Major Cardiac Defects', *Ultrasound in Obstetrics and Gynecology*, 10: 242–6.

Lou, S., Dahl, K., Risör, M. B., Hvidman, L. E., Thomsen, S. G., Jörgensen, F. S., Olesen, F., Kjaergaard, H. and Kesmodel, U. (2007) 'En kvalitativ undersøgelse av gravides valg av nakkefoldscanning (A Qualitative Study of Pregnant Women's Choice of an NT-Scan)', *Ugeskriftet for Laeger* (*Danish Medical Journal*), 169: 914–18.

Lundeby, H. and Tøssebro, J. (2007) 'Family Structure in Norwegian Families of Children with Disabilities', *Journal of Applied Research in Intellectual Disabilities* (OnlineEarly Articles), doi: 10.1111/j.1468–3148.2007.00398.x.

Hall, S., Bobrow, M. and Marteau, T. M. (2000) 'Psychological Consequences for Parents of False Negative Results on Prenatal Screening for Down's Syndrome: Retrospective Interview Study', *British Medical Journal*, 320: 407–12.

Müller, M. A., Bleker, O. P., Bonsel, G. J. and Bilardo, C. M. (2006) 'Nuchal Translucency Screening and Anxiety Levels in Pregnancy and Puerperium', *Ultrasound in Obstetrics and Gynecology*, 27: 357–61.

Nicolaides, K. H., Azar, G., Byrne D., Mansur, C. and Marks, K. (1992) 'Fetal Nuchal Translucency: Ultrasound Screening for Chromosomal Defects in First Trimester of Pregnancy', *British Medical Journal*, 304: 867–9.

NRK (2007) Bare Marte, Faktor, NRK1. Available HTTP: < http://sesam.no/search/?c = wt&q = %22bare+marte%22# > (accessed 12 March 2007).

NTB (1999) 'Ultralyd-stopp ved RiT (Ultrasound Study Stopped at the Hospital in Trond-heim)', *Nasjonal Telegram Byraa*, 15 October.

Öhman, S. G., Saltvedt, S., Grunewald, C. and Waldenström, U. (2004) 'Does Fetal Screening Affect Women's Worries About the Health of Their Baby?', *Acta Obstetricia et Gynecologica Scandinavia*, 83: 634–40.

Öhman, S. G., Saltvedt, S., Waldenström, U., Grunewald, C. and Olin-Lauritzen, S. (2004) 'Pregnant Women's Response to Information About an Increased Risk of Carrying a Baby with Down Syndrome', *Birth*, 33: 64–73.

Press, N. (2000) 'Assessing the Expressive Character of Prenatal Testing: The Choices Made or the Choices Made Available?', in E. Parens and A. Asch (eds), *Prenatal Testing and Disability Rights*, Washington, DC: Georgetown University Press.

Saetnan, A. R. (2000) 'Thirteen Women's Narratives of Pregnancy, Ultrasound and Self', in A. R. Saetnan, N. Oudshoorn and N. Kirejczyk (eds) *Bodies of Technology: Women's Involvement with Reproductive Medicine*. Columbus, OH: Ohio State University Press.

Shakespeare, T. (2006) *Disability Rights and Wrongs*, London and New York: Routledge.

Singer, P. (1994) *Rethinking Life and Death: The Collapse of Our Traditional Ethics*, Oxford: Oxford University Press.

Skotko, B. (2005) 'Mothers of Children with Down Syndrome Reflect on Their Postnatal Support', *Pediatrics*, 115: 64–77.

Skovmand, K. (2005) 'Flere kræver erstatning etter fejlscanning (More and More Claim Compensation for Wrongful Birth)', *Politiken*, 11 October.

Spencer, K., Souter, V., Tul, N., Snijders, R. and Nicolaides, K. H. (1999) 'A Screening Program for Trisomy 21 at 10–14 Weeks Using Fetal Nuchal Translucency, Maternal Serum Free-Human Chorionic Gonadotropin and Pregnancy-Associated Plasma Protein-A', *Ultrasound in Obstetrics and Gynecology*, 13: 231–7.

Stainton, T. (2003) 'Identity, Difference and the Ethical Politics of Prenatal Testing', *Journal of Intellectual Disability Research*, 47: 533–9.

Sundhedsstyrelsen (Danish Ministry of Health) (2003) *Fosterdiagnostik og risikovurdering: rapport fra en arbeijdsgruppe* ('Prenatal Diagnosis and Risk Assessment – a Report'), Copenhagen: Sundhedsstyrelsen.

Taipale, P., Hiilesmaa, V., Salonen, R. and Ylöstalo, P. (1997) 'Increased Nuchal Translucency As a Marker for Fetal Chromosomal Defects', *New England Journal of Medicine*, 337: 1654–8.

Taylor, C. (1995) 'The Politics of Recognition', in C. Taylor (ed.), *Philosophical Arguments*, Cambridge, MA: Harvard University Press.

Vehmas, S. (2002) 'Parental Responsibility and the Morality of Selective Abortion', *Ethical Theory and Moral Practice*, 5: 463–84.

13   Biopolitics and bare life

Does the impaired body provide contemporary examples of *homo sacer?*

Donna Reeve

Introduction

Whilst the work of the Italian philosopher Giorgio Agamben has been applied within disciplines such as sociology, political science and even geography, it has yet to be fully embraced by disability studies. In *Homo Sacer* (1998), Agamben explores the nature of sovereign power and production of bare life, describing *homo sacer* as someone whose 'entire existence is reduced to a bare life stripped of every right by virtue of the fact that anyone can kill him without committing homicide' (Agamben 1998: 183).

Homo sacer can be considered to be an outlaw or bandit who lives in a state of exception, someone who is not simply outside the law and indifferent to it, but who has instead been abandoned by the law. Whilst Agamben uses *homo sacer* to analyse global conflict and politics, I will utilise this figure on a less grand scale to present several ideas about how *homo sacer* can provide a model for some contemporary examples of disablism.

I have applied Agamben's work to a diverse set of issues affecting disabled people within the UK. First, I will show that prenatal diagnosis can provide clear examples of bare life within which 'normative schemes of intelligibility establish what will and will not be human, what will be a liveable life, what will be a grievable death' (Butler 2004: 146). I will then explore the ways in which the contentious issue of enforced psychiatric hospitalisation of people with severe mental distress can be linked to recent discussions about the nature of refugee camps and detention centres – examples of modern-day 'camps' that represent states of exception. Finally, I will use the concept of *homo sacer* to consider some examples of psycho-emotional disablism arising from interactions with strangers. If practices such as staring or name-calling happen when behavioural norms or 'internal laws' are suspended, then disabled people with visible impairments can end up feeling disempowered within what is effectively a *psychic*, rather than spatial state of exception.

This chapter aims to show that Agamben's concepts of states of exception and the figure of *homo sacer* have some relevance to the experience of people with impairments within contemporary UK society. Whilst I am not suggesting that disabled people are outlaws forced to live outside of society in the same ways as refugees or detainees, nonetheless an analysis of some aspects of disablism through the lens of Agamben still has value for disability studies as well as for the wider academic field.

Biopolitics: the figure of *homo sacer*

It was Foucault who first coined the term 'biopolitics' to describe the manner in which sovereignty was replaced by an active interest in the well-being of citizens. Foucault suggested that biopolitics had two poles. First, starting in the seventeenth century, disciplinary powers emerged which acted at the level of the individual body (such as prisons and work houses). This was then followed at a later point by bio-power which operated on the species body whose 'supervision was effected through an entire series of interventions and *regulatory controls: a bio-politics of the population*' (ibid.: 139, italics in original). Thus the emergence of biopolitics marked the end of sovereign power, 'cut[ting] off the king's head' (Foucault 2004: 59) and instead locating power within systems of knowledge and social apparatuses. Through this new productive power operating at the biological level, Foucault revealed how biopolitics was vital to the creation of a capitalist society which relied on the socialisation of the body to provide labour power (Foucault 2000a).

In contrast, Agamben (1998) argues that biopolitics has been in existence since ancient times and deliberately conflates sovereignty and biopolitics. Agamben draws on an obscure figure of archaic Roman law, *homo sacer*, to illustrate the essential part played by bare life within modern politics. *homo sacer* is someone 'who *may be killed and yet not sacrificed*' (Agamben 1998: 8, italics in original); thus the killing of *homo sacer* is not considered to be homicide. In addition: 'He who has been banned is not, in fact, simply set outside the law and made indifferent to it but rather *abandoned* by it, that is, exposed and threatened on the threshold in which life and law, outside and inside, become indistinguishable' (ibid.: 28, italics in original).

This zone of indistinction represents a state of exception in which *homo sacer* is bare life, *zoē*, stripped of political rights and located outside the *polis* (city); in other words *homo sacer* has biological life, but that life has no political significance. Additionally the act of abandonment cleaves the biological (*zoē*) and the social/political (*bios*) and provides the route by which biological life is included within the realm of power (Diken and Laustsen 2005: 20). The spatial and psychic zones of exception evident within the experience of disablism will provide examples of this act of abandonment.

As well as the relationship between *homo sacer* and zones of exception, Agamben shows that there is a reciprocal relationship between the sovereign and *homo sacer*: 'the sovereign is the one with respect to whom all men are potentially *homines sacri*, and *homo sacer* is the one with respect to whom all men act as sovereigns' (Agamben 1998: 84). Diken and Laustsen (2005) argue that academic scholars usually focus attention on the first part of the formulation, possibly because of the misguided association between the sovereign and the state and thereby maintain the illusion of indivisibility. This ends up blocking the insights offered by the second part which describes the relationship between *homo sacer* and other people; I will show the importance of this latter relationship when understanding the experience of psycho-emotional disablism.

Homo sacer has existed in different guises at different points in time. For example, in medieval times witches could be seen as *homines sacri* (Diken and Laustsen 2005). Trials of women who were claimed to be witches were held in local courts who suspended the usual procedural rules; therefore witches were included and excluded from the law simultaneously. Agamben (1998) discusses at length the example of Jews in Nazi Germany who had their citizenship revoked and who were then transported to concentration camps where millions died. The concentration camp was an example of a state of exception in which the citizen became *homo sacer*, bare life, 'life unworthy of being lived' (ibid.: 142). The atrocities carried out in these camps were made possible by the way in which Jews, as well as other minority groups such as homosexuals, Gypsies and disabled people, were viewed as less than human. Agamben concludes that whilst the events in Germany were extreme, it is the camp which is the fundamental biopolitical paradigm of Western society (ibid.: 181). This concept of the 'camp' has been applied to more contemporary examples such as the 'non-places' which contain detainees or refugees (Diken and Laustsen 2005). Although these are not places where people can be justifiably killed, there are analogies in the ways in which people find themselves abandoned by the law, living as *homo sacer* in a zone of indistinction, neither included or excluded. In particular, much attention has been paid to the case of Camp Delta where 'detainees' (rather than 'prisoners') exist in a state of exception because of their ambiguous legal status. President Bush issued a military order that authorised the 'indefinite detention' of non-citizens suspected of being terrorists. These people are not POWs as defined by the Geneva Convention; the camp is situated in Guantánamo Bay which is outside the borders of the US, on Cuban soil, but outside the realm of Cuban law (Butler 2004; Diken and Laustsen 2005). Therefore these detainees represent examples of *homo sacer* because they are at the mercy of presidential decrees and the will of military personnel.

The shadowy figure of *homo sacer* would likewise seem to be a valuable metaphor for the impaired figure, especially given the ways in which people such as professionals and even the general public can act as 'sovereign' towards disabled people. Within social theory, Agamben is regarded as a philosopher who has developed the ideas of Foucault to explain contemporary political phenomena. Given the amount of literature which has been devoted to applying Foucault to issues of health, impairment and disability, it is surprising that the work of Agamben has not been likewise utilised to date; this chapter aims to start to rectify this omission.

Disability definitions

Before discussing some examples of the application of *homo sacer* to issues affecting disabled people, it is important that I explain my definitions of disability. Within UK disability studies, disability is viewed as a form of social oppression experienced by people with impairments. Disablism can be considered to be analogous to racism, sexism, ageism and homophobia, experiences of social discrimination, exclusion and even violence towards people who are marked out as 'different'. In her recent book Thomas (2007) amends her earlier social relational understanding of *disability* (Thomas 1999) to instead refer to *disablism*. Thus 'disablism is a form of social oppression involving the social imposition of restrictions of activity on people with impairments and the socially engendered undermining of their psycho-emotional well-being' (Thomas 2007: 115).

This word shift is an attempt to make clear the connection between disability and social oppression rather than limitations in activity (impairment effects). The use of the term 'disablism' ensures that discussions about the different forms of social oppression experienced by people with impairments remains in the realm of the social relational (rather than with the individual) and can be easily related to the sister terms of racism, sexism and ageism which people are generally more familiar with.

Disablism operates along two different pathways. The 'restrictions of activity' refer to the structural dimensions of disablism which are barriers which affect what people can *do*; for example environmental restrictions which prevent people with impairments physically accessing buildings and social spaces. The second pathway refers to the psycho-emotional dimensions of disablism which are barriers that undermine people's psycho-emotional well-being, affecting who they can *be*; for example, dealing with the thoughtless comments or stares of strangers which can leave someone with a visible impairment feeling psychologically and emotionally undermined. Whilst disability studies has been excellent at theorising the structural dimensions of disablism, the psycho-emotional dimensions remain relatively understudied (Reeve 2004; Thomas 1999). It should also be noted that the experience of psycho-emotional disablism is not an inevitable consequence of being impaired (a medical model view) or a 'private trouble' which distracts from the real battles against a disabling society (Thomas 2007).

As commented earlier, there are many examples of Foucauldian approaches to disability theory and practice (see, for example, Allan 1996; Chadwick 1996; Corker and French 1999; Hughes and Paterson 1997; Hughes 1999; McIntosh 2002; Price and Shildrick 1998; Reeve 2002; Sullivan and Munford 1998; Tremain 2005). However there is a scarcity of examples where the work of Agamben has been applied to disability studies (see, for example, Overboe 2007; Sirnes 2005). In this chapter I will expand the application of Agamben's work to three very different areas within UK disability studies: prenatal diagnosis, proposed changes to the Mental Health Act and one example of psycho-emotional disablism arising from interactions between disabled people and strangers. Finally, I will discuss the potential value of *homo sacer* and states of exception in helping to understand contemporary experiences of disablism.

Prenatal diagnosis

In his book on *homo sacer*, Agamben discusses the controversy surrounding the blurred area between death and brain stem death (BSD) as well as the concept of 'neomort', a body with the legal status of a corpse, but kept alive to allow the harvesting of organs for transplant (Agamben 1998). These are contemporary examples of *homo sacer*, bare life; another is that of prenatal diagnosis and abortion (Sirnes 2005). The issue of prenatal diagnosis is a highly emotive and contested area – it is seen by many disabled activists and academics as an attempt to detect and then eliminate disabled babies. In my view Shakespeare (2006a) presents a well-balanced discussion of prenatal diagnosis and concludes that it is not deliberately eugenic or simply discriminatory as some would claim.

However, one area that does need reform is current abortion law in the UK which prohibits termination after the twenty-fourth week of pregnancy, except in cases where there is a substantial risk that the child would be born with severe physical or mental impairments (Shakespeare 1998). Thus there is no time limit for the possible termination of a severely impaired foetus – abortion is authorised up to and even during birth. This loophole in the law was intended to cover the very few cases where the foetus was unlikely to survive to birth, or to die soon after. However, as the law does not give a definition of 'seriously handicapped', it is left up to the discretion of parents, doctors and a host of other professionals to decide where the line should be drawn, who in effect then act as sovereign to the foetus. This has resulted in cases where late abortions have taken place where impairment was not severe enough to cause the neonatal death of the infant – notoriously the example of two foetuses with cleft palate, a condition which is not life-threatening in itself (Day 2003).

In addition, maternity and screening services have become increasingly routinised; as a result, prenatal diagnosis becomes the norm (rather than the exception) and women ask less questions about the implications of the screening (Reist 2005). The relationship between prenatal testing and late abortion is downplayed to encourage women to accept the test (Markens *et al.* 1999). If impairment, such as Downs Syndrome or spina bifida, is detected after twenty-four weeks, then the lack of good quality, balanced information about the impairment means that late termination of the impaired foetus is often seen as the only option (Shakespeare 2006a). The failure of the law to clearly define which impairments are serious enough to consider late abortion for the affected foetus causes a range of sovereign decisions, each one of which will be influenced by the attitudes and behaviour of medical professionals as well as larger cultural attitudes held about disability.

Sirnes (2005) provides a thorough analysis of this state of exception where the disabled foetus could be considered to be *homo sacer*, both inside and outside the law. Sirnes argues that there is a 'double insecurity' present; not only are evaluations being made about where the foetus lies on the abnormal/normal continuum, but what is considered to be 'normal' today, may be considered 'abnormal' in the future. Finally, this blurred area of the law with the vague reference to 'serious handicap' is not simply about the killing of a human being without legal punishment; as well as the question of whether the foetus can be considered to be a human being, there is also the issue of the status afforded to the potential infant. The non-disabled foetus has an expectation of a 'political life' whereas this is far less certain for the disabled foetus, who, by the very interpellation of being labelled as disabled, becomes abjectified (Overboe 2007).

Compulsory detention of people with severe mental distress

The work of Agamben has been applied to many examples of contemporary residential 'camps' such as refugee camps, detention centres as well as gated communities – housing complexes offering high levels of security and protection for residents, designed to keep people out rather than in (Diken and Laustsen 2005). I will now examine the contentious issue of detaining people with severe mental distress in psychiatric hospitals and show how this can lead to a state of exception. The term 'severe mental distress' is being used here in preference to 'severe mental health problems' in line with the development of a social model of madness and distress which directly challenges individual models of mental health (Beresford 2002). Currently there are plans to strengthen the mental health law in the UK which would allow people with untreatable mental health conditions, such as severe personality disorders to be detained even if they have not committed a crime (BBC News 2006). Under the current law, someone with a psychopathic disorder can only be forcibly detained, for the protection of themselves or others, if their condition is treatable. In addition the amendments include extending the use of compulsory treatment outside hospital to patients living in the community which could include the setting of curfews on these patients, or what have been termed 'psychiatric Asbos' (Batty 2006). This Bill is being opposed by backbench MPs and campaigners because it gives the authorities the power to restrict people's civil liberties and ironically is likely to deter some vulnerable and potentially dangerous people from seeking treatment in the first place. A press release from the British Medical Association Medical Ethics Committee stated that:

> It is essential that anyone with a mental health disorder can only be compulsorily treated if there is some clear health benefit linked to this action. Mental health legislation cannot be used to detain people whom the authorities simply want locked away. If people are deemed a danger to others then criminal proceedings need to be implemented, if appropriate.
>
> (Calland 2006)

Thus someone with severe mental distress could lose the protection typically afforded to people by criminal law (innocent until proven guilty) and instead find themselves entangled within mental health law which legitimately restricts their human and civil rights.

> By law, mental health service users' rights can be removed in the name of 'treatment'. They can be subjected forcibly to 'treatments' which are evidenced to have damaging, sometimes fatal, effects – treatments which include

neurosurgery, electro-convulsive treatment (ECT) and the use of outdated and risky psychotropic/neuroleptic drugs.

(Beresford *et al.* 2002: 389–90)

Therefore once someone has been detained under the Mental Health Act they can be subject to treatment; whilst there will be cases where this is highly appropriate and/or desirable for the person in question, others will experience treatment which in other circumstances would be seen as a form of assault. It is at this point that a state of exception exists because these people find themselves in hospital, with greatly reduced human and civil rights and being forcibly 'treated'. What would normally be considered abusive is allowed within this setting and patients can become *homo sacer*, subject to the 'sovereign' power of the doctors, social workers and other professionals who control their daily life, treatment and release date. Additionally, the very nature of the reason for their incarceration means that any attempts at protestation or resistance are likely to be seen as further proof of their need for treatment.

Government mental health policy currently sees people with severe mental distress as 'dangerous', feels the need to ensure 'public safety' as a priority and then is justified in achieving this through an emphasis on control and 'compulsory' treatment (both in hospital and within the community) (Beresford 2004: 247). This has uncomfortable echoes with the current rhetoric about the 'war on terror' and the increasing number of anti-terrorism bills being legislated here in the UK; the Queen's Speech in November 2006 contained the eighth anti-terrorism Bill since Prime Minister Blair came to power in 1997 (Jones 2006). I mentioned earlier the descriptions of Camp Delta and the ways in which it represented a state of exception with the detainees being bare life or *homo sacer*. One of the precedents which the US Government has used to support the detention of people without criminal charge has been the involuntary hospitalisation of people with severe mental distress who pose a threat to themselves or others (Butler 2004). The increasing panic and fear about the threat from terrorism is leaking into other areas of public life such as the treatment of people with severe mental distress which simply feeds prejudice about the assumed threat posed by this group of people to the population at large. Being 'seen' as dangerous for whatever reason can lead to indefinite detention (Butler 2004).

Interactions with strangers

Prenatal diagnosis and the forced treatment of people with severe mental distress represent examples of the first part of the symmetrical relationship between the sovereign and *homo sacer*: 'the sovereign is the one with respect to whom all men are potentially *homines sacri*' (Agamben 1998: 84; italics in original). They are examples of structural disablism where decisions made by professionals or politicians (sovereign) result in the exclusion of people with impairments from mainstream life either through incarceration or *in extremis*, through not being born. I now want to reframe Agamben's concept of the state of exception to look at examples of psycho-emotional disablism which represent examples of the second part of the relationship: '*homo sacer* is the one with respect to whom all men act as sovereigns' (ibid.: 84; italics in original).

The reactions of people, particularly strangers, towards people with visible impairments can have a detrimental effect on emotional well-being and can indirectly restrict what disabled people *do*: 'It is not only physical limitations that restrict us to our homes and those whom we know. It is the knowledge that each entry into the public world will be dominated by stares, by condescension, by pity and by hostility' (Morris 1991: 25).

The experience of being stared at or called names can be emotionally draining (Keith 1996); additionally it is not just the encounter itself that is disabling, but the 'existential insecurity' associated with the uncertainty of not knowing how the next stranger will react further compounds this example of psycho-emotional disablism (see Thomas 2004: 38 for more discussion about existential security). As one disabled woman wrote:

> But more than the occasional pointing finger or tactless word, it is the not knowing which is unnerving. To know that I make an impression on anyone who sees me, and yet (thanks to the convention of politeness), do not know what impression, is unsettling. Am I just mildly odd and worth only a moment's extra appraisal? Or am I a freak – tolerated and capable of commanding affection, but a freak all the same?
>
> (Satyamurti 2001: 52)

This extract reveals how Satyamurti feels continually at risk of being abandoned as a freak. In addition, Satyamurti describes her difficulties about how she should think of *herself* as disabled: 'If I give up disputing the obvious and fully acknowledge my physical difference, will I be buried alive in a box labelled "invalid?"' (ibid.: 53). Again there is this theme of being 'put' somewhere else, of being abandoned by those she meets.

According to Agamben, it is the act of abandonment which separates out those that are considered to be political beings (citizens, *bios*) from bare life (biological bodies, *zoë*) (Agamben 1998). This leaves *homo sacer* as bare life, outside the *polis*, and like Girard's scapegoat 'not protected by norms and rules, which apply to others, and being considered of no worth' (Diken and Laustsen 2005: 21). If one considers the manner in which disabled people can end up being labelled as a freak or invalid by others, then it could be suggested that disabled people are placed in a *psychic* state of exception. In the spatial states of exception, such as refugee camps and detention centres, it is juridical law that is suspended; in the case of these psychic states of exception it is 'norms' of behaviour which are suspended, 'internal laws', which leave disabled people feeling outside of 'mainstream society', different to others.

For example, in the UK it is generally considered rude to stare, but nonetheless disabled people with visible impairments/impairment effects are often stared at,

beyond what could be considered the point of polite curiosity. This act of objectification has the effect of marking a person with impairments as a non-person,
thereby moving them into a different psychic space to the observer. Part of being
seen as a non-person means that it is assumed that the impaired person doesn't
mind being imitated, called names or avoided – that unlike most non-disabled
people, they are not hurt, offended or upset by such experiences. This is particularly true for people with learning difficulties who are perceived as being
incapable of feeling emotions such as shame, embarrassment or upset, because
of the nature of their impairment (Marks 1999). It is telling that in the UK,
although incitement to racial hatred was made illegal in 1965, hate crimes
against disabled people only became illegal in April 2005 – forty years later
(Quarmby 2007).

Methods of objectification move with the times. Shakespeare (2006b) describes
the experience of being a victim of 'camera abuse', an everyday occurrence since
mobile phones with an inbuilt camera became commonplace:

> And somehow, while it's always unpleasant to be the subject of intrusive
> attention, it feels even more disempowering to be captured on camera phone.
> There's no possible answer to that click which could make it better. Making
> a rude response only shows that the perpetrators have succeeded in getting
> under your skin. There's no point in complaining to the police, because unless
> the photo is published, then no crime has been committed. If you smash their
> phone, then you become the criminal.
>
> (Shakespeare 2006b)

I would regard this form of 'camera abuse' as another example of psycho-emotional
disablism, one which is very difficult to challenge or prevent. Shakespeare would
argue that it is inevitable that people will always stare at him because no amount
of education will eliminate this 'natural curiosity' – rather than being a form of
oppression, being stared at is one of the 'dimensions of my predicament as a dwarf'
(Shakespeare 2006a: 63). However, whilst curiosity may be part of human nature,
being captured on camera phone is far more objectifying and should be treated as
unacceptable behaviour.

It is at the point of these direct person–person interactions that the ontological
insecurity of *homo sacer* is most clearly revealed. By its very nature psycho-
emotional disablism usually manifests within a relationship between two people,
and so a disabled person, like *homo sacer* is subject somewhat to the 'goodwill' of
others within this encounter – people can act as sovereign to the disabled person,
either including them or placing them in this ambiguous psychic state of exception. I use the term 'goodwill' reservedly; ignorance plays a big part in many
social encounters as there is a lack of culturally 'agreed' rules of engagement
(Keith 1996: 72). All too often fear of 'doing the wrong thing' results in avoidance
rather than engagement.

Discussion

I have provided some examples of how Agamben's work, in particular his use of the figure of *homo sacer* moving within the state of exception represented by a 'camp', can be applied to the experiences of disabled people. In addition to showing how juridical laws around mental health and abortion in the UK can give rise to 'spatial' states of exception, I have suggested that the suspension of 'moral' laws can similarly lead to 'psychic' states of exception. However, Agamben is not without his critics. One major criticism is that his work is too apocalyptic (Bull 2004) and paints an image where there is no escape from the camp. For example, in the case of Camp Delta, the detainee is only freed when President Bush revokes the 'state of emergency' or a military tribunal takes place – both are sovereign actions. Foucault wrote about the interconnection between power and knowledge and suggested that resistance emerges because of the existence of power and in opposition to it (Foucault 2000b). Resistance can exist because there is something to push against and challenge such as normalising discourses. However, Agamben describes a situation which is far more uncertain and precarious, in which chaos is normal and the exception has become the rule. Therefore resistance is a much more slippery concept here simply because there is nothing tangible which can be resisted. The only possible alternative to this would be a form of 'escape' from the camp, which provides an opportunity for 'something other' (Diken and Laustsen 2005: 13), the possibility of a creative line of escape.

For disabled people, where pragmatic solutions to the problems associated with living in a disabling society are required, this looks like a dead end theoretically. If Foucauldian approaches, like post-structuralism generally, have been criticised for their inability to make a difference to the material disadvantage associated with disablism (Thomas 1999), then Agamben would appear to offer even less to disability studies. However, the world we live in is becoming more uncertain and fragmented and this affects disabled people as well as others in society. In a recent article in a grassroots magazine, Mike Oliver and Colin Barnes discussed the problems facing the disabled people's movement at the start of the twenty-first century (Oliver and Barnes 2006). They concluded that focusing on disability as a rights issue will not remove disablism and will only benefit a small minority of disabled people: 'At worst, it will legitimise further the rhetoric of those who support an inherently unjust and inequitable society and hamper further the struggle for meaningful equality and justice' (ibid.: 12).

For these two writers, the growing professionalisation of disability rights and the gradual closures of organisations of disabled people such as centres for independent/integrated living (CILs) has contributed to the decline of the disabled people's movement. The Government has adopted 'social model speak' but has failed to improve significantly the life of many disabled people (Prime Minister's Strategy Unit 2005). As far as the general population are concerned, disabled people are protected by anti-discrimination law, the Disability Discrimination Act. However, terms like 'reasonable adjustment' mean that exclusion is still the reality for some disabled people; but it can be difficult to continue protesting about exclusion when others assume the 'problem' has gone away because ramps and disabled parking spaces are now more commonplace. Therefore disabled people live in an age where inclusion and exclusion can and do coexist in many areas of their lives and it is becoming increasingly difficult to challenge disablism effectively. Thus the work of Agamben can be applied to the current situation we find ourselves in, if only to understand the effects of the slippery usage of social model terminology by the government and other public bodies.

Agamben also describes how every society, however modern, decides who its *homo sacer* is, whose life is seen as 'life devoid of value' (Agamben 1998: 139). Recent proposed changes to the welfare system include the moving of one million disabled people off incapacity benefits and into some form of paid employment (Preston 2006). This emphasis on employment as the only appropriate route out of poverty has led to the concern that those disabled people who are unable to work because of their impairment/impairment effects will:

> feel 'written off' and of no value because they are not able to work. Disabled people need a decent income (so comprehensive benefits advice is crucial), good social and health care, as well as access to education, and training, in order to play their full part in society according to their abilities. *Non-workers should not be written off as non-citizens.*

> (Reith 2005: 8; my emphasis)

Thus disabled people who are unable to work could end up being seen as non-citizens just like *homo sacer*, as bare life (*zoē*) outside the *polis*.

I have offered some starting suggestions as to how the ideas of Agamben might be applied to the experience of disablism and whilst some useful insights can be gained, it is not easy to see how successful escape attempts might be made from some of the states of exception I discussed earlier. In the case of prenatal diagnosis the law needs to be changed (a sovereign decision) to ensure that late termination is only allowed in cases where the life of the mother is at risk or if the foetus will die before birth or during the first twenty-eight days of life (Shakespeare 2006a); the state of exception will then disappear. In addition, prospective parents need much more accurate information about what it means to have a disabled child so that they make an informed choice about the fate of an impaired foetus (ibid.). Parents who then decide to continue with the pregnancy provide the escape route for the impaired foetus by allowing him or her to be born. Similarly it will be down to legal processes to ensure that people experiencing severe mental distress do not become subject to 'indefinite detention'.

However, creative lines of escape are far more feasible if one considers the psychic states of exception I discussed earlier. In part this is because one is dealing with informal, conventional 'rules' of behaviour rather than juridical laws. In the example of interaction with strangers, I discussed how people with visible impairments can be left feeling invalidated and vulnerable when stared at by others, or when asked intrusive questions. One solution to this problem will come with time – the 'rules of engagement' with disabled people will become more widely known and accepted as disabled people become more visible in society, supported by the gradual erosion of disablist images and prejudices. Inclusion in schools will produce future generations of people who are accustomed to having disabled friends and colleagues. However, in the short term, lines of escape can be observed as individual disabled people find ways of dealing in a creative way with the prejudices of others. For example, some will take on the role of being an educator, showing the other person that disabled people do not need to be feared (Reeve 2006). This does take effort and a certain amount of emotion work on the part of the disabled person to help the other person 'deal with *their* fears and prejudices [about disability]' (Reeve 2006: 104). Whilst this should not be necessary, it does smooth the social interaction and has the potentially altruistic outcome in easing future interactions between that person and other disabled people. It also returns control to the disabled person over the social encounter and they can then move out of the state of exception and back into the social world, effectively returning *zoē* to the *polis*.

Conclusion

I have used the work of Agamben, drawing on his concepts of *homo sacer* and states of exception, to consider various examples of structural and psycho-emotional disablism. These reveal contemporary states of exception – spatial and psychic – which provides a valuable description of the increasingly uncertain, contradictory and fragmented world that disabled people can find themselves in. Foucauldian approaches have been useful in understanding the technologies of power which differentiate the normal from the abnormal; the focus on the suspension of law and production of exception described by Foucault's student Agamben offers additional insight into the uncertain world which many disabled people face in the UK, and elsewhere, at the start of the twenty-first century. In particular I have introduced the concept of psychic states of exception to explore psycho-emotional disablism within interpersonal interactions, in which others act as sovereign to the disabled person, their attitudes and actions either including or excluding *homo sacer* from the mainstream.

The bodies of *homines sacri* are all around us – in addition to the well-documented figures of the refugee and political detainee, I would include the impaired foetus, the person with severe mental distress, the disabled person experiencing hate crime. The consequences of longer life expectancies in Western societies means that more people will experience impairment at some point in their life – anyone can become disabled. Thus the continual 'taken-for-granted non-impaired body' represents a theoretical oversight in this post-structural turn where uncertainty and difference are fundamental considerations in contemporary social theory about the body. Whilst there is an interest in theoretical figures such as cyborgs and monsters, no connection is made between these figures and the lived experience of disabled people (Garland-Thomson 2005). As well as applying Agamben's ideas within disability studies, it is vital that the lived experience of disabled people becomes part of the mainstream of social theory with the impaired body being acknowledged as providing yet more examples of contemporary *homo sacer*.

Bibliography

Agamben, G. (1998) *Homo Sacer: Sovereign Power and Bare Life*, trans. D. Heller-Roazen, Stanford, CA: Stanford University Press.

Allan, J. (1996) 'Foucault and Special Educational Needs: A "Box of Tools" for Analysing Children's Experiences of Mainstreaming', *Disability and Society*, 11: 219–33.

Batty, D. (2006) 'Mental Health Sector Criticises 'Unworkable' Reforms', Online. Available HTTP: < http://www.guardian.co.uk/medicine/story/0,1950763,00.html > (accessed 21 November 2006).

BBC News (2006) 'Plan to Beef Up Mental Health Law', Online. Available HTTP: < http://news.bbc.co.uk/go/pr/fr/-/1/hi/health/6157736.stm > (accessed 20 November 2006).

Beresford, P. (2002) 'Thinking About "Mental Health": Towards a Social Model', *Journal of Mental Health*, 11: 581–4.

—— (2004) 'Treatment at the Hands of the Professionals', in J. Swain, S. French, C. Barnes and C. Thomas (eds), *Disabling Barriers: Enabling Environments*, 2nd edn, London: Sage Publications.

Beresford, P., Harrison, C. and Wilson, A. (2002) 'Mental Health Service Users and Disability: Implications for Future Strategies', *Policy Press*, 30: 387–96.

Bull, M. (2004) 'States Don't Really Mind Their Citizens Dying (Provided They Don't All Do It at Once): They Just Don't Like Anyone Else to Kill Them', Online. Available HTTP: < http://www.generation-online.org/p/fpagamben2.htm > (accessed 25 May 2005).

Butler, J. (2004) *Precarious Life: The Powers of Mourning and Violence*, London: Verso.

Calland, T. (2006) 'BMA Response to the Queen's Speech – Proposed Mental Health Legislation Refers to England and Wales Only', Online. Available HTTP: < http://www.bma.org.uk/pressrel.nsf/wlu/SGOY-6VKGC5?OpenDocument&vw = wfmms > (accessed 21 November 2006).

Chadwick, A. (1996) 'Knowledge, Power and the Disability Discrimination Bill', *Disability and Society*, 11: 25–40.

Corker, M. and French, S. (eds) (1999) *Disability Discourse*, Buckingham: Open University Press.

Day, E. (2003) 'The Law Is Saying There Are Reasons Why I Shouldn't Be Alive. I Look at My Life and Think: That's Rubbish', *The Sunday Telegraph*, 23 November, p. 22.

Diken, B. and Laustsen, C. B. (2005) *The Culture of Exception: Sociology Facing the Camp*, London and New York: Routledge.

Foucault, M. (1990) *The History of Sexuality: Volume 1, An Introduction*, trans. R. Hurley, New York: Vintage Books.

—— (2000a) 'The Birth of Social Medicine', in J. D. Faubion (ed.), *Michel Foucault, Essential Works: Vol. III: Power*, trans. R. Hurley, New York: The New Press.

—— (2000b) 'The Ethics of the Concern for Self as a Practice of Freedom', in P. Rabinow (ed.), *Michel Foucault, Essential Works: Vol. I: Ethics*, trans. P. Aranov and D. McGrawth, London: Penguin Books.

—— (2004) *'Society Must Be Defended': Lectures at the Collège de France, 1975–76*, trans. D. Macey, London: Penguin Books.

Garland-Thomson, R. (2005) 'Feminist Disability Studies', *Signs*, 30: 1557–87.

Hughes, B. and Paterson, K. (1997) 'The Social Model of Disability and the Disappearing Body: Towards a Sociology of Impairment', *Disability and Society*, 12: 325–40.

Hughes, B. (1999) 'The Constitution of Impairment: Modernity and the Aesthetic of Oppression', *Disability and Society*, 14: 155–72.

Jones, G. (2006) 'Queen's Speech Focuses on Security', Online. Available HTTP: < http://www.telegraph.co.uk/news/main.jhtml?xml=/news/2006/11/15/uelizabeth115.xml > (accessed 22 November 2006).

Keith, L. (1996) 'Encounters with Strangers: The Public's Responses to Disabled Women and How This Affects Our Sense of Self', in J. Morris (ed.), *Encounters With Strangers: Feminism and Disability*, London: Women's Press.

Markens, S., *et al.* (1999) '"Because of the Risks": How US Pregnant Women Account for Refusing Prenatal Screening', *Social Science and Medicine*, 49: 359–69.

Marks, D. (1999) *Disability: Controversial Debates and Psychosocial Perspectives*, London and New York: Routledge.

McIntosh, P. (2002) 'An Archi-Texture of Learning Disability Services: The Use of Michel Foucault', *Disability and Society*, 17: 65–79.

Morris, J. (1991) *Pride Against Prejudice: Transforming Attitudes to Disability*, London: Women's Press.

Oliver, M. and Barnes, C. (2006) 'Disability Politics and the Disability Movement in Britain: Where Did It All Go Wrong?', *Coalition* (August): 8–13.

Overboe, J. (2007) 'Disability and Genetics: Affirming the Bare Life (the State of Exception)', *Canadian Review of Sociology and Anthropology*, 44: 219–35.

Preston, G. (2006) 'Introduction', in G. Preston (ed.), *A Route Out of Poverty? Disabled People, Work and Welfare Reform*, London: Child Poverty Action Group.

Price, J. and Shildrick, M. (1998) 'Uncertain Thoughts on the Dis/Abled Body', in M. Shildrick and J. Price (eds), *Vital Signs: Feminist Reconfigurations of the Bio/logical Body*, Edinburgh: Edinburgh University Press.

Prime Minister's Strategy Unit (2005) 'Improving the Life Chances of Disabled People', Online. Available HTTP: < http://www.strategy.gov.uk/downloads/work_areas/disability/disability_report/pdf/disability.pdf > (accessed 31 July 2006).

Quarmby, K. (2007) 'If These Are Not Hate Crimes, What Are?', *Disability Now* (September): 1.

Reeve, D. (2002) 'Negotiating Psycho-Emotional Dimensions of Disability and Their Influence on Identity Constructions', *Disability and Society*, 17: 493–508.

—— (2004) 'Psycho-Emotional Dimensions of Disability and the Social Model', in C. Barnes and G. Mercer (eds), *Implementing the Social Model of Disability: Theory and Research*, Leeds: The Disability Press.

—— (2006) 'Towards a Psychology of Disability: The Emotional Effects of Living in a Disabling Society', in D. Goodley and R. Lawthom (eds), *Disability and Psychology: Critical Introductions and Reflections*, Basingstoke: Palgrave.

Reist, M. T. (2005) 'Introduction', in M. T. Reist (ed.), *Defiant Birth: Women Who Resist Medical Eugenics*, Melbourne: Spinifex Press.

Reith, L. (2005) 'Disability Alliance Response R47: Response to the Work and Pensions Committee Inquiry into the Reform of Incapacity Benefits and Pathways to Work', Online. Available HTTP: < http://www.disabilityalliance.org/r47.pdf > (accessed 6 August 2006).

Satyamurti, E. (2001) 'The Seamstress', *Prospect* (February): 52–3.

Shakespeare, T. (1998) 'Choices and Rights: Eugenics, Genetics and Disability Equality', *Disability and Society*, 13: 665–81.

—— (2006a) *Disability Rights and Wrongs*, London and New York: Routledge.

—— (2006b) 'Snap Unhappy', Online. Available HTTP: < http://www.bbc.co.uk/ouch/columnists/tom/290806_index.shtml > (accessed 27 September 2006).

Sirnes, T. (2005) 'Deviance or homo sacer? Foucault, Agamben and Foetal Diagnostics', *Scandinavian Journal of Disability Research*, 7: 206–19.

Sullivan, M. and Munford, R. (1998) 'The Articulation of Theory and Practice: Critique and Resistance in Aotearoa New Zealand', *Disability and Society*, 13: 183–98.

Thomas, C. (1999) *Female Forms: Experiencing and Understanding Disability*, Buckingham: Open University Press.

—— (2004) 'Developing the Social Relational in the Social Model of Disability: A Theoretical Agenda', in C. Barnes and G. Mercer (eds), *Implementing the Social Model of Disability: Theory and Research*, Leeds: The Disability Press.

—— (2007) *Sociologies of Disability and Illness: Contested Ideas in Disability Studies and Medical Sociology*, Basingstoke: Palgrave Macmillan.

Tremain, S. (ed.) (2005) *Foucault and the Government of Disability*, Ann Arbor, MI: University of Michigan Press.

Index

Numbers in *italics* denote tables

Parfit, D. 116
part-essentialist individual deficiency interpretation (PEID) 17, 18, 20, 21, 22, 23
paternalism 3, 9
Paterson, K. and Hughes, B. 43
peer interaction: and language acquisition 145, 147–8; and signed language 148
perception 61
persistent vegetative state 172, 180 n5
personhood 6, 77, 78–80; and children 82; claim of psychological personhood 83, 86, 90 n15, 90 n22; descriptive 88 n3; Feinberg on 88 n3; institutional status concept of 79, 88, 89 n5; normative 88 n3; psychological concept of 78–9, 82–3; status concepts of 79, 87–8, 88 n3; *see also* interpersonal personhood
phantom limb sensation 71 n9
phenomenology 5, 58–9; and variation 65–6; *see also* Merleau-Ponty, M.
philosophy 3
Pogge, T. W. 96–8, 102 n6, 112
political philosophy 6
politics 51–2
politics of disablement interpretation (POD) 15, 18, 19, 20, 22, 23, 24, 27
power 4, 17–18, 44, 51, 52, 174, 212; political 127–8, 130; *see also* autonomy; sovereign, the
pre-implantation genetic diagnosis (PGD) 154
prejudice 109, 174, 209
prenatal diagnosis 9, 203, 207–8, 209, 213; *see also* prenatal screening
Prenatal Diagnosis and Risk Assessment (Sundhedsstyrelsen) 185–6
prenatal screening 9, 33, 49; arguments against 188; and autonomy 185–6, 187, 193–5; challenges 195–8; Denmark 194, 196; disability discussion 198; Down syndrome 185–200; good-maternal-care discussion 198–9; Norway 187–8, 193, 194; as offensive 189–90, 192–3; *see also* prenatal diagnosis
Press, N. 188
Pride Against Prejudice (Morris) 22–3
psychiatric diagnosis 49–51
psycho-emotional disablism 10, 206, 210, 214; and camera abuse 211; *homo sacer* as 211; staring as 210–11; as state of exception 210–11
psychological concept of personhood and

recognitive attitudes 82–3
psychopathy 90 n22
quality adjusted life years (QALYS) 169
quality of life (QL) 58; assessment of 177–9, 179–80; doctors as experts 173–5; dominance of medical profession 175–6; and law 169; medical assessments unchallenged 176–7; and medical model of disability 171–3
Quinn, M. 39

Rawls, J. 6, 93; theory of justice 93, 95, 96, 98, 102 n5, 112; worth of liberty 93, 95–6, 97–8, 99
realisable freedom 99–100
Re C 178, 182 n53
recognitive attitudes 77, 80–1, 89 n3; and psychological concept of personhood 82–3
reification 45, 90
Reith, L. 213
Re J 173–4
respect 81, 82
rights 87, 90 n23; A-C-rights 139; A-rights 139; C-rights 140, 143, 149; *see also* disability rights movement; open future; women's rights movement
right to language 137, 138, 150; and open future 143–6
right to life 79, 88 n3

Satyamurti, E. 210
Savulescu, J. 160, 165
Schiavo, T. 59, 70 n2
Searle, J. 5, 47
self, the 27; *see also* identity
Sellars, W. 79, 89 n5
Sen, A. 84–5, 103 n9, 116–17
severe mental distress 213; and compulsory detention 208–9; and *homo sacer* 209
Shakespeare, T. 106, 131, 188–9, 194, 207, 211
Silvers, A. 106, 111
Sirnes, T. 207
Skjervheim, H. 140
social arrangements 4, 42, 100
social construct: disability as 44–5, 54 n1, 128, 159; women as 128
social constructionism 42, 44–5, 52
social construction of disablement interpretation (SCOD) 20–1, 22, 23–4, 25, 26, 27